WITHDRAWN
May be sold for the benefit of
The Branch Libraries of The New York Public Library
or donated to other public service organizations.

The GI Made Simple

THE PROVEN WAY TO LOSE WEIGHT, BOOST ENERGY AND CUT YOUR RISK OF DISEASE

Sherry Torkos B.Sc. Phm.

D1308093

⊗WILEY

John Wiley & Sons Canada, Ltd.

Copyright © 2007 by Sherry Torkos

All rights reserved. No part of this work covered by the copyright herein may be reproduced or used in any form or by any means—graphic, electronic or mechanical—without the prior written permission of the publisher. Any request for photocopying, recording, taping or information storage and retrieval systems of any part of this book shall be directed in writing to The Canadian Copyright Licensing Agency (Access Copyright). For an Access Copyright license, visit www.accesscopyright.ca or call toll free 1-800-893-5777.

Care has been taken to trace ownership of copyright material contained in this book. The publisher will gladly receive any information that will enable them to rectify any reference or credit line in subsequent editions.

Library and Archives Canada Cataloguing in Publication Data

Torkos, Sherry

    The GI made simple : the proven way to lose weight, boost energy and cut your risk of disease / Sherry Torkos.

Includes bibliographical references.
ISBN 978-0-470-15415-1

    1. Glycemic index. 2. Reducing diets. I. Title.
RM222.2.T669 2007   613.2'5   C2007-905538-9

Production Credits
Cover design: Ian Koo
Cover photography: Stockbyte
Interior text design: Tegan Wallace & Jason Vandenberg
Printer: Quebecor – Fairfield

John Wiley & Sons Canada, Ltd.
6045 Freemont Blvd.
Mississauga, Ontario
L5R 4J3

Printed in the United States of America

1 2 3 4 5 QW 11 10 09 08 07

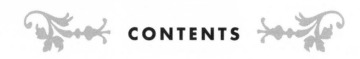 **CONTENTS**

I dedicate this book to everyone who is interested in improving their health and having greater energy and well-being. It is my sincere hope that this book empowers you on your journey to optimum health.

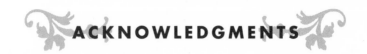

ACKNOWLEDGMENTS

There are many people I would like to acknowledge and thank for their help with this book.

My husband Rick for all your support and encouragement throughout this book project and all the others over the years.

To my developmental editor Kate Zia, I can't thank you enough for your guidance and assistance with all aspects of this book. It is a pleasure working with you.

To the team at John Wiley & Sons: Christiane Cote, Leah Fairbank, Liz McCurdy, Jennifer Smith, and Valerie Ahwee, I thank you for this opportunity, and your literary guidance and expertise throughout the process.

A special thanks to my colleagues Mitch Skop, Dean Mosca, Tom McCartney, and Mike Danielson for all your support in this book and the many other projects that we have worked on together.

Thanks to Johanna Burani, MS, RD, CDE, Jennifer O'Callaghan, and Saul Katz for reviewing this manuscript and providing suggestions.

I would also like to acknowledge the many researchers that have worked so hard to help us understand obesity, weight loss, and the role of glycemic control: Thomas Wolever, DM, PhD; David J.A. Jenkins, MD; Jenny Brand-Miller, PhD, DSc; Harry Preuss, MD; and Jay Udani, MD.

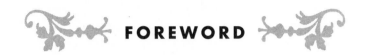# FOREWORD

$\mathcal{B}$y now, most of us understand that being overweight is not just an appearance issue, or about the inconvenience of having many different clothing sizes in your closet. As a medical practitioner; professor of physiology, medicine and pathology; and researcher in the field of obesity and weight loss, I can attest to obesity's power to destroy one's health and quality of life—both mentally and physically.

It is generally recognized that being obese predisposes an individual to diabetes mellitus, coronary artery disease, stroke, sleep apnea, degenerative joint disease, and most likely certain forms of cancer. In January 2004, the *Journal of Obesity Research* published a study co-authored by the US Centres for Disease Control that estimated that American obesity-attributable medical expenditures reached $75 billion in 2003 and that taxpayers financed about half of these costs through Medicare and Medicaid. Therefore, I applaud Sherry's commitment to educating the public about this very serious health issue. Clearly we must take action if we want to live well.

While many fad diets promise miraculous results, unfortunately far too many are based on hype rather than science. Dietary changes are critical, but there are other factors to consider. A balanced approach to weight loss includes several lifestyle modifications in addition to dietary regimens—exercise (both aerobic and anaerobic), avoidance of stress, and adequate sleep. This book pulls it all together and appeals not only to those trying to lose weight but also to those interested in improving their health and cutting their risk of chronic disease.

A low glycemic diet that lessens the load of rapidly absorbed carbohydrates is a healthy way of eating, because it is associated with better blood sugar control, superior health, and improved weight management. Like the majority of North Americans, I love good food, and I can confirm that an eating style that improves the glycemic load is not restrictive or hard to follow. It incorporates reasonable portions of fresh, whole, unprocessed foods that possess healthful nutrients.

Why worry about rapidly rising blood sugar concentrations? Too much sugar rising in the circulation from poor dietary choices is associated with insulin resistance, which can lead to all sorts of health problems, including diabetes. Accordingly, controlling rapid elevations in blood sugar can reduce your risk of several chronic diseases, and even slow the advance of symptoms associated with aging. Gaining control of your blood sugar also helps reduce appetite and cravings for sweets, and enhances energy levels.

The glycemic index and the glycemic load are new tools that help us understand how carbohydrates impact blood sugar. It is worth repeating that numerous studies have linked diets high in the glycemic load to obesity and increased risk factors for heart disease, diabetes and cancer. On the other hand, low glycemic index and load diets have been shown to help protect against these conditions.

This book will help you make the transition to better health by educating you on the rationale behind the glycemic index and glycemic load for weight loss and overall health, teaching you how to make healthy low glycemic food choices, and giving you simple strategies for incorporating a low glycemic diet into your daily life. You will also find information on other factors that influence weight, and advice on how to improve these aspects of your life. From advice on supplements that can help improve blood sugar control and aid weight loss to tips on making adjustments in all aspects of your life, Sherry empowers you to make the necessary lifestyle changes that will enable you to live a higher quality of life.

Harry Preuss, MD, MACN, CNS, is a tenured professor at Georgetown Medical Center. His current research centers on the use of dietary supplements and nutraceuticals to favorably influence or even prevent obesity, insulin resistance, and heart disease. The author of hundreds of medical papers and abstracts, he is co-author of The Prostate Cure *(Crown, 1998) and the new book* The Natural Fat-Loss Pharmacy *(Broadway, 2007). He lives in Fairfax Station, Virginia.*

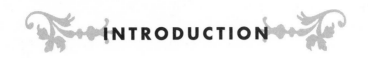

INTRODUCTION

$\mathscr{C}$hances are that this book caught your eye because you've struggled to lose weight and heard that the glycemic index was the latest diet phenomenon. It is true that the glycemic index, or GI, is certainly getting a lot of attention, but the story of the glycemic index is not about the latest diet touted by celebrities; it's a scientifically supported way of eating. The GI is about making good food choices that will improve blood sugar regulation and ultimately yield long-term health benefits. In fact, if you're looking for a diet that only provides rapid weight loss, I'm afraid you've got the wrong book. Following a low-glycemic diet has been shown to reduce weight and body fat, but the GI diet is not another quick fix.

Eating according to the glycemic index is based on science and physiology, and is geared for those who are willing to commit to their lifelong health. It is for those people who want to learn about the profound effects of blood sugar imbalances, and want to take action before those imbalances turn into chronic disease. So, this is not simply another diet book. If you take the time to learn about the glycemic index, and make the necessary changes to your diet and lifestyle, you will be amazed with the results. While you may not have found the quick-fix diet you thought you wanted, you did find the healthy diet you need to reach your weight-loss goals and improve your overall health: The glycemic index is the ideal tool to help you succeed.

The Glycemic Index: Short and Sweet

First introduced in the 1980s by Canadian researchers, the glycemic index is a system of ranking all forms of carbohydrates (from breads to vegetables) on a scale of zero to 100 on how they affect blood glucose levels and consequently insulin levels. If a carbohydrate is digested quickly and causes a rapid rise in blood sugar levels, it is considered to be high GI. If a carbohydrate is more slowly digested and causes a gentle rise in blood sugar levels, it is considered low GI. Research indicates that eating carbohydrates that are low GI *as well as healthy* (very important!) can help support weight loss and decrease body fat. This way of eating will also improve blood sugar regulation, which in turn will help balance mood, reduce hunger cravings and appetite, and increase metabolic rate—all important factors to promote long-term weight loss. Plus, a low-GI diet has been found to reduce the risk of diabetes and heart disease, which are two of the biggest health threats we face today.

Is the Glycemic Index Right for Me?

The glycemic index is not a diet in the typical sense of that word. It is a way of eating that involves making healthy carbohydrate choices. If you follow a low-GI diet, you will still eat a balanced and varied selection of carbohydrates, along with quality proteins and healthy fats. There are no food-combining rules to memorize, no calorie counting, and no depriving yourself of a particular food group. Your food consumption is not restricted beyond eating healthy portion sizes, and there are absolutely no missed meals. The glycemic index can be followed by people of all ages, and does not cause any adverse effects, like some fad diets. Even people with existing health concerns, such as type 2 diabetes and heart disease, can follow a low-glycemic diet. In fact, there are significant health benefits to eating according to the glycemic index because it not only helps combat obesity and diabetes, two conditions at nearly epidemic proportions, but also addresses a growing health concern today: insulin resistance.

How to Use this Book: Just the Facts, Please

I've written this book to provide you with a thorough explanation of the role of the glycemic index in weight loss, disease prevention, and optimal health. I've made the science as reader-friendly as possible, using the latest research and providing the best resources for you to refer to.

I start the book with a quick overview of the worldwide obesity epidemic and its impact on your health. I discuss the problems associated with fad diets and our obsession with weight. I explain the causes of obesity and factors affecting body weight and provide information on how to determine your ideal weight.

In Chapter 2 you'll find a complete description of the glycemic index and gain an understanding of why the medical community is underscoring the importance of choosing low-glycemic carbohydrates.

Chapter 3 discusses the role of insulin in blood sugar management and how insulin resistance leads to diabetes and metabolic syndrome. You will learn about how blood sugar and insulin affect appetite, mood, fat storage, aging, heart health, and sexual function.

Finding dietary balance with your carbohydrates, proteins, and fats is discussed in Chapter 4. Here you will get the basics on these necessary food groups and learn how to make quality choices without compromising taste or enjoyment.

Chapter 5 covers the role of exercise, sleep, and stress management for glycemic control, weight loss, disease prevention, and more. Find out what types of exercises to do and how much you need to get the best results—you'll be surprised! You will also learn how stress and lack of sleep affect hormones that are involved in body weight regulation and get great tips for reducing stress and improving sleep.

In Chapter 6 you get my recommendations as a pharmacist on nutritional supplements that can help improve blood sugar control and support weight loss. I have reviewed the science on these products and provide you with a summary of the benefits and appropriate use of these products.

Lastly, in Chapter 7, you'll roll up your sleeves, take what you've learned, and put it into action. I have my top 10 list of dietary strategies, a glycemic index food values chart, tips on satisfying snacks, stocking your pantry, eating out, and surviving the holidays. You'll also find two weeks of meal recommendations to get you started in the right direction.

The Glycemic Index Is Here to Stay

The glycemic index has only recently received the attention and recognition that it deserves. What has propelled the glycemic index to the forefront of the fields of nutrition and weight loss is the fact that it is scientifically based ... and, quite simply, it works! Over 20 years of clinical research conducted around the world have validated the glycemic index as a tool that can safely and effectively promote weight loss, improve blood sugar and insulin levels, and control appetite and cravings. Following a low-glycemic diet can also help lower risk factors for heart disease. Plus, following a low-glycemic diet will give you more physical and mental energy. With all these health benefits, it is not surprising that this way of eating has gained acceptance among doctors, dietitians, and other health care professionals.

Unlike many of the fad diets, following a low-GI diet is not restrictive or hard to follow. It is easy, flexible, and satisfying. It is a healthful way of eating that is here to stay. In this book I have put together the most up-to-date information on the glycemic index and made it simple for you to understand and follow. I am confident that you are going to enjoy the health benefits of following this new way of eating, so let's get started!

1
THE OBESITY EPIDEMIC

 Our society is bombarded by a tremendous amount of information on research and developments in the area of lifestyle, fitness, and nutrition, yet we're slow to put that good information into action in our lives. Around the world, our lifestyles are increasing our risk of heart disease, diabetes, and other chronic diseases, yet until we are diagnosed, many of us don't feel motivated to make changes in our daily habits. Experts agree these diseases are largely preventable; however, heart disease remains the number one killer of men and women in Western societies; diabetes impacts an estimated two million Canadians and 21 million Americans; and osteoarthritis is predicted to become a leading cause of disability within the next decade. This apathy toward our long-term health is nowhere more apparent than when it comes to weight and the global obesity epidemic. Consider this stunning statistic: *Around the world an estimated one billion people are classified as either overweight or obese.*

Change is not easy, especially when it comes to lifestyle factors such as diet and exercise. With our fast-paced way of living, priorities get waylaid and we don't take time for sleep, proper eating, and regular exercise, which are all required for a healthy body. Sadly, despite the attention given to the obesity epidemic, we are not making much progress. Rates are continuing to soar, affecting younger and younger people, and bringing on chronic diseases and premature death.

Startling Statistics

Currently, in the United States over 60 percent of adults are overweight, with 30 percent classified as obese. These figures represent an increase of more than 50 percent in just one decade. Direct medical costs are an astounding $105 billion or 9 percent of the nation's health care costs.

In Canada, obesity rates are up in almost every age group, with a notable increase among children and adolescents. According to the 2004 Canadian Community Health Survey, 8 percent of children ages 12–17 are obese, compared to 3 percent in the 1978/79 survey. In the same time frame, adult obesity rates nearly doubled from 14 percent to 23 percent; that represents 5.5 million Canadians struggling not just with excess weight, but also with obesity. This health epidemic translates into an estimated $5 billion burden on the Canadian economy. And while men and women are equally likely to be obese, the survey found a higher percentage of women in the most severe category of obesity, significantly increasing their risk of developing chronic diseases. Sadly, statistics indicate that obese individuals have a 50–100 percent likelihood of dying prematurely due to chronic disease caused by obesity.

The Global Perspective

It is estimated that there are over 300 million obese people worldwide. Despite the attention given to this health crisis, rates are continuing to soar everywhere. The United Kingdom, Australia, New Zealand, Canada, and Mexico all report obesity rates of over 20 percent. Here is a quick look at the situation in some of the heaviest countries:

> ❧ In the United Kingdom, obesity rates have quadrupled in 25 years, with *three-quarters of the population overweight* and an estimated 22 percent classed as obese. The childhood obesity rate has tripled in 20 years. Over 30,000 deaths are attributed to obesity, costing the nation over £7 billion per year in health care and related costs.

- In Australia, *obesity rates have more than doubled* in 20 years, with approximately 48 percent of the population classified as overweight or obese.

- In New Zealand, *one-third of the adult population is overweight and one-fifth of the adult population is obese,* according to a New Zealand Ministry of Health report in 2003.

- In Mexico, obesity rates are one of the highest in the world, with over *60 percent of adults overweight or obese in 1999* (up from 33 percent in 1988). One report indicated that obesity rates might rise to as high as 85 percent for women and 75 percent for men.

- While overall obesity rates in China, Japan, Korea, and other Asian countries are much lower, they have been steadily climbing. In fact, the rate of *obesity in China has tripled* in five years, and is as high as 20 percent in some urban cities.

Childhood Obesity

Sadly, young people are the largest growing segment of the obese population. According to an estimate by the International Obesity Task Force, 22 million of the world's children five years and younger are overweight or obese. A study conducted by the California Department of Health Services, found that 80 percent of children have been on a diet by the time they have reached the fourth grade. In the United States, child obesity rates have almost tripled in 25 years. The picture is worse in Canada. A long-term study of Canadian children revealed that at least one in four are overweight. Unfortunately, this trend is also being seen in other areas of the world such as Europe, Australia, and the Caribbean.

The obesity epidemic is having far-reaching effects on the health of our children. A recent study found one in eight children have three or more risk factors for metabolic syndrome, a cluster of symptoms that serve as an early warning signal for heart disease and diabetes. And more than half of these children have at least one risk factor. These risk factors include high blood pressure, inefficient processing of glucose, elevated insulin levels, low levels of "good" HDL cholesterol, and elevated triglycerides.

Overweight children are at risk of becoming obese adults, and obese adults are at greater risk for raising obese children. While genetics are often blamed, in many cases it is poor lifestyle habits that are learned or "inherited" rather than faulty genes.

Research Spotlight:
"Children Developing Pot-Bellies"

Led by researchers at the US Centers for Disease Control, a recent study published in *Pediatrics* reports that abdominal obesity in American children increased more than 65 percent among boys and almost 70 percent among girls between 1988 and 2004. This was startling news because studies have shown that the increased risk of heart disease and type 2 diabetes due to excess body fat is mainly due to belly fat. While the study reported an overall increase in body mass index in children from youngsters to teens, what worried experts was the significant increase in abdominal or belly fat. The good news is that, for children and adolescents, the negative health effects from excess belly fat are often reversible through changes to diet and lifestyle.

Obesity's Impact on Health

It is hard to escape the warnings from our national health agencies. The message they deliver is clear: *Obesity increases the risk of developing chronic disease.* Obesity is one of the most preventable causes of chronic disease because in most cases its development is lifestyle-related. Taking in too many calories, eating unhealthy foods, and not getting enough exercise are poor lifestyle choices that can lead to serious consequences. These are not the only factors that affect our weight, but they are the major ones. Some of the other elements that affect body weight are discussed in a later section of this book.

> Obesity's impact is so diverse and extreme that it should now be regarded as one of the greatest neglected public health problems of our time, with an impact on health which may well prove to be as great as that of smoking. —World Health Organization

The Heart of the Matter

One of the most serious consequences of being overweight is the increased risk of heart disease. Carrying excess weight increases blood pressure because the heart has to work harder and becomes strained. Having elevated blood pressure, known as hypertension, increases the risk of coronary heart disease and stroke.

Those who are overweight also tend to develop high cholesterol and there are several reasons for this. First, eating a diet high in saturated and trans fats can raise cholesterol levels. Second, overweight individuals are at risk for developing insulin resistance, a condition where the body becomes resistant to the effects of insulin so that insulin and blood sugar levels remain high. When insulin levels are high, the liver increases triglyceride production, which lowers HDL (good) cholesterol and increases LDL (bad) cholesterol. This combination of factors can substantially increase the risk of heart disease.

Obesity and Cancer

According to the US National Cancer Institute, obesity and physical inactivity may account for 25–30 percent of several major cancers—colon, breast (postmenopausal), endometrial, kidney, and esophagus. Some studies have also reported links between obesity and cancers of the gallbladder, ovaries, and pancreas.

There are several reasons why obesity increases cancer risk. With respect to colon cancer, high levels of insulin or insulin-related growth factors in obese people are believed to promote tumor development. For breast cancer, the risk appears to be tied to the higher levels of estrogen. After menopause, estrogen is produced in the fat tissue. Obese women have greater fat tissue and can produce higher amounts of estrogen, which can stimulate the growth of estrogen-sensitive tissues. Obese women are also at greater risk of dying from breast cancer because tumors are more difficult to detect and thus the women are diagnosed at a later stage of cancer.

Diabesity: The Union of Obesity and Diabetes

One of the most talked about consequences of obesity is the development of diabetes. Researchers have ever coined a name for this association: "diabesity." According to a report from the Centers for Disease Control, diabetes has officially reached epidemic proportions. Obesity reduces insulin sensitivity, causing a problem called insulin resistance, which is the precursor to type 2 diabetes. The link between obesity and diabetes is quite strong—over 80 percent of people with type 2 diabetes are overweight or obese. Researchers agree that the more weight you carry, the greater your chances of suffering from diabetes and other blood sugar-related conditions.

Other health risks associated with obesity include postsurgical complications, delayed wound healing, and an increased risk of infection and gout. Excess weight can put pressure on your lungs and chest, making it difficult to breathe and causing sleep apnea. It can be stressful to the joints, back, and hips, leading to osteoarthritis, limited mobility, pain, and discomfort. Overweight and obese women are also at greater risk of experiencing infertility and complications during childbirth.

What's Lifestyle Got to Do with It?

It seems to go without saying that the likelihood of being overweight or obese is related to diet and exercise. According to the 2004 Canadian Community Health Survey, adult men and women who ate fruit and vegetables less than three times a day were more likely to be obese than were those who consumed such foods five or more times a day. This is not surprising because when unhealthy foods (fast foods, processed foods) take the place of healthy foods (such as fruits and vegetables), calorie intake increases and blood sugar regulation is impaired, both of which cause weight gain. Similarly, people who were sedentary rather than physically active were more likely to be obese: 27 percent of sedentary men were obese, compared with 20 percent of active men. Among women, obesity rates were high not only for those who were sedentary, but also for those who were moderately active. The message is simple: We must learn how to eat a healthy, balanced diet, and lead active lifestyles.

Desperately Dieting

The prevalence of obesity is a paradox in our thinness-obsessed Western culture. As a result, North Americans spend billions in an effort to slim down. It is estimated that North Americans spend more than $46 billion annually on weight-loss products and services. Weight Watchers, established in 1961, now has annual sales of over $1 billion. There are endless programs, products, and diet pills on the market. It is estimated that more than $6 billion is spent yearly on diet pills alone. The concern here is that many of these products do not work. Very few diet pills have been clinically tested, and some may even be hazardous to your health. And when dieters do lose weight, they usually gain it back. Studies show that one year after dieting, 66 percent of people regain any lost weight. Government findings report that after five years, *97 percent of dieters regained all the weight they had lost.* Maintaining weight loss is even more difficult than losing it because it takes a long-term commitment to a lifestyle that involves healthy eating and regular exercise. Slipping back to old habits is hard to resist.

Fad Diets Are Not the Answer

Despite the failure and frustration of fad diets, we get enticed by the sensational advertisements and are keen to hear about and try the newest weight-loss miracle. Each week there seems to be a new diet program or plan promoted in the tabloids. Promises for quick results and celebrity endorsements give us false hope and the belief that these plans will work for us. Unfortunately, many of these diets are not backed by science, and some can be dangerous to your health. For example, a diet I recently came across promotes that you can lose 10 pounds in two days by consuming a liquid tonic of various herbs and nutrients. No food is allowed, or any liquids other than water for the two days. It is important to realize that rapid weight loss that occurs from fasting or taking diuretics and laxatives is temporary and can be dangerous, especially for those with diabetes, or kidney or heart problems. Once you start eating and drinking fluids again, the weight will come back.

Stay away from diets that are drastically low in calories (less than 800 calories per day). While these diets can lead to rapid weight loss, they are not without risks. Low-calorie diets cause the body to cannibalize (break down) its own muscle for fuel, causing muscle-wasting, which reduces metabolism. Plus, these diets can cause nutrient deficiencies, fatigue, reduce immune function, and, over the long term, may result in more serious consequences such as organ failure.

Are You Overweight or Obese?

Most of us realize when we gain weight: Our pants get tighter, we have to extend our belts, or we hop on the scale and see the numbers go up. But how much weight gain is too much? At what point does that weight gain become dangerous? There are a variety of methods that doctors and medical professionals use to determine whether your weight or fat gain could be putting you at risk of developing health problems.

Body Mass Index

The BMI is the easiest and most commonly used screening tool. It is an internationally accepted mathematical formula that is highly correlated with health risk, meaning the higher the number, the greater the risk of developing consequences such as heart disease and diabetes.

The BMI takes into consideration your height and weight and provides ranges that are considered normal, overweight, and obese. The BMI is calculated by taking your weight in kilograms and dividing it by your height in meters squared. Check the chart on the following page to find your BMI. Here is how you calculate it using imperial measurements:

1. Multiply your weight, in pounds, by 0.45
2. Multiply your height, in inches, by 0.025
3. Square the answer from step 2
4. Divide the answer from step 1 by the answer from step 3

BMI (kg/m2)	19	20	21	22	23	24	25	26	27	28	29	30	35	40
Height (inches)	Weight (pounds)													
58	91	96	100	105	110	115	119	124	129	134	138	143	167	191
59	94	99	104	109	114	119	124	128	133	138	143	148	173	198
60	97	102	107	112	118	123	128	133	138	143	148	153	179	204
61	100	106	111	116	122	127	132	137	143	148	153	158	185	211
62	104	109	115	120	126	131	136	142	147	153	158	164	191	218
63	107	113	118	124	130	135	141	146	152	158	163	169	197	225
64	110	116	122	128	134	140	145	151	157	163	169	174	204	232
65	114	120	126	132	138	144	150	156	162	168	174	180	210	240
66	118	124	130	136	142	148	155	161	167	173	179	186	216	247
67	121	127	134	140	146	153	159	166	172	178	185	191	223	255
68	125	131	138	144	151	158	164	181	177	184	190	197	230	262
69	128	131	142	149	155	162	169	176	182	189	196	203	236	270
70	132	139	146	153	160	167	174	181	188	195	202	207	243	278
71	136	143	150	157	165	172	179	186	193	200	208	215	250	286
72	140	147	154	162	169	177	184	191	199	206	213	221	258	294
73	144	151	159	166	174	182	189	197	204	212	219	227	265	302
74	148	155	163	171	179	186	194	202	210	218	225	233	272	311
75	152	160	168	176	184	192	200	208	216	224	232	240	279	319
76	156	167	172	180	189	197	205	213	221	230	238	246	287	328

If your BMI is under 18.5, you may be underweight. If your BMI falls between 18.5 and 24.9 your weight is likely within normal range. If your BMI is over 25, you are probably overweight. If it is over 30, you are likely obese. There are a few drawbacks with the BMI. It does not distinguish fat from lean body mass (muscle, bone, and tissue). For example, a professional bodybuilder could appear to be obese using the BMI. It also doesn't take into account the higher body fat content normally found in females.

Body Fat Check

Body composition (the amount of fat versus muscle) is a much more important factor in determining health risk than just looking at overall body weight. There are several ways to check your body fat percentage, including:

- *Bioelectric Impedance:* A machine is used to measure an electric signal as it passes through lean body mass and fat. The higher the fat content, the greater the resistance to the current.

- *Near Infrared Technology:* Infrared light is shone onto the skin (usually the bicep area). Fat absorbs the light, while lean body mass reflects the light back. The reflected light is measured by a special sensor, transmitted into the computer, and translated into percentage of body fat. This method is highly accurate and is available at health centers and gyms.

- *Dual Energy X-ray Absorptiometry (DEXA):* X-ray energies are used to measure body fat, muscle, and bone mineral. This method is highly accurate but also the most expensive and time consuming.

Men with more than 25 percent and women with more than 30 percent body fat are considered to be obese. The target body fat range for women is 15–25 percent, and for men it is 10–20 percent.

Apples versus Pears: Where's Your Fat?

Researchers have discovered that it's not just how much extra body fat a person carries, but where the fat is stored on the body that increases the risk of disease. People who carry excess fat around their middle (apple-shaped body), are more likely to develop serious health problems (such as type 2 diabetes, high cholesterol and blood pressure, coronary heart disease, and stroke) than people who store their excess fat in their hips and thighs (pear-shaped body).

Abdominal or "visceral" fat indicates that there is excess fat surrounding the internal organs. This fat is associated with greater health risks because it produces various hormones and chemicals that can trigger inflammation, insulin resistance, and other deleterious health effects. Excess belly fat is recognized as a significant risk factor for a condition called *metabolic syndrome*, which greatly increases one's risk of type 2 diabetes and heart disease. Aside from belly fat, signs of metabolic syndrome include elevated blood pressure, high triglycerides, insulin resistance, and low levels of HDL cholesterol ("good" cholesterol).

Abdominal obesity is influenced by a number of factors, including genetics and lifestyle choices. Regular physical activity, not smoking, and using unsaturated fat over saturated fat have been shown to decrease the risk of developing abdominal obesity.

> To determine whether your waist is putting you at risk, take out a tape measure and put it around your waist just above the navel. A waist circumference of more than 40 inches (102 cm) for men or more than 35 inches (89 cm) for women is associated with a substantially increased risk of developing disease.

Factors That Contribute to Obesity

In the past, it was thought that weight gain was the result of taking in more energy (food) than you expend (exercise/activity). Conversely, reducing food intake and increasing exercise was believed to be the key to weight loss. For years, doctors and researchers believed this simple theory to be the answer. We now know, however, that many other factors can contribute to weight gain. Some people can exercise religiously, reduce food intake, and still not lose weight. And, of course, we all know people who can eat whatever they want and never gain weight. Weight gain and obesity are complex matters, dependent upon various lifestyle, hormonal, biochemical, metabolic, and genetic factors. Here are some of the most important factors that affect our weight and ability to store or burn fat.

Basal Metabolic Rate (BMR)
Your BMR is the rate at which your body burns calories at rest. This rate is dependent on several factors, such as activity level and thyroid function. Having a sluggish metabolism means that your body burns calories more slowly, and this is represented by a low BMR.

Caloric Intake
Overeating and consuming more calories than your body uses for energy can result in weight gain, regardless of whether those calories come from fat, carbohydrates, or protein. Excess calories that are consumed and not burned for energy are stored by the body in the form of fat.

Physical Activity
Our activity level is a major player in weight balance. Inactivity causes loss of muscle mass, a reduced metabolic rate, and increased body fat. Conversely, regular exercise can improve muscle mass and boost metabolism. As we exercise, our muscles utilize calories for energy and generate heat, which promotes the burning of fat.

Quality of Food
Eating poor-quality foods—such as foods high in saturated fat, sugar, and refined, processed and fast foods—is associated with weight gain.

These foods are energy dense (high in calories). They can also trigger hormone and blood sugar imbalances, which are associated with weight gain and inability to lose weight. Food quality is just as important as food quantity.

Stress

Chronic stress, which is common today, is a major contributor to weight gain. Stress increases the production and release of cortisol, a hormone that promotes fat storage, particularly around the midsection (belly). Stress comes in many forms, not just from our outside environment (work, family, finances). For example, eating high-glycemic foods triggers a quick and strong surge in insulin levels, which is stressful to the body and increases the release of cortisol.

Lack of Sleep

Getting too little sleep (less than six hours per night), even for as short a period as a week, can trigger hormonal imbalances such as decreased sensitivity to insulin, decreased production of leptin and serotonin, and increased levels of a hormone called ghrelin, all factors that trigger increased appetite and fat storage. Lack of sleep also reduces human growth hormone production, which can slow down your metabolism.

Genetics

Genetics is commonly blamed for obesity. It is true that we inherit our genetic code from our parents, and we have no control over certain characteristics, such as our bone structure and height. However, we also inherit our diet and lifestyle habits from our parents, and experts agree that having a genetic predisposition toward obesity does not mean that this is your destiny. Several studies have shown that lifestyle factors are more important determinants of obesity and these factors can also switch the obesity genes on or off.

Hormones and Brain Chemicals

- **Insulin:** Insulin is the hormone secreted by the pancreas, which regulates blood sugar levels. When insulin levels are high, the body stores more fat and is not able to use fat as a source of energy. This is the reason insulin is also known as "the fat-storage hormone." High insulin levels result from eating high-GI foods and having insulin resistance, which is discussed later in this book.

- **Thyroid:** The thyroid gland plays a vital role in controlling metabolism. If your thyroid levels are low (hypothyroidism), this can reduce your metabolic rate and cause weight gain. This is a very common cause of weight gain, especially in women ages 30–50 years, and can develop from chronic stress, or autoimmune disease. Symptoms of low thyroid include fatigue, hair loss, dry skin, constipation, low libido, and sensitivity to cold.

- **Leptin:** Satiety (a feeling of fullness) is partly regulated by leptin, a hormone produced by body fat. Researchers have found that some people become resistant to their own leptin. To compensate for this, the body produces more and more of the hormone, but the brain does not properly receive the "satisfied" message.

- **Serotonin:** Serotonin is a chemical messenger in the brain that also regulates satiety. When levels are low, we feel hungry and when they are high, we feel satisfied. Serotonin levels are lower in people who suffer from depression. Stress and high cortisol levels can also lower serotonin levels. Certain weight-loss products elevate serotonin to promote satiety and reduce cravings for food.

- **Human Growth Hormone (HGH):** By increasing lean muscle mass and reducing body fat storage, human growth hormone regulates body weight. Levels decline with age, particularly after age 50, causing a shift in our body composition. As HGH decreases, we gain body fat and lose muscle mass.

✦ **Estrogen:** High estrogen levels are associated with weight gain. Estrogen is produced by the ovaries before menopause. Many women find that they gain weight after menopause because, as ovaries slow down, the fat cells take over the production of estrogen. In order to meet the growing demand during menopause, the fat cells increase in size and number. Estrogen levels are also higher in women taking birth control pills and those with poor liver function because the liver is responsible for detoxifying and processing estrogen. We also get estrogen from the environment (plastics, pesticides, and certain cosmetics). Men also produce some estrogen, and those with high body fat have higher estrogen levels, which can cause growth of the breasts and belly.

✦ **Testosterone:** Testosterone helps the body maintain lean muscle mass and burn fat. A deficiency of this hormone can cause a loss of muscle mass and a fat gain. Testosterone levels decline with age and this is a significant contributor to fat gain in older men.

Lose Weight and Live Longer

Controlling your weight may extend your lifespan. In a study published in the *Journal of the American Medical Association*, researchers looked at body weight and mortality in a group of 19,000 middle-aged men over the course of 27 years. Researchers found that the men who were lean lived significantly longer than those who were extremely under- or overweight. This is no surprise, considering the effects that excess weight has on your risk of developing chronic life-shortening diseases.

Research among women has yielded similar results. A study published in the May 2004 issue of the *Journal of the American Medical Association* found that both obesity and physical activity significantly and independently affected mortality. This study involved over 115,000 women who were followed for 24 years. Compared to physically active, lean women, there was nearly a two-and-a-half-fold increase in risk of death for inactive and obese women. The researchers estimated that excess weight (BMI over 25) and physical inactivity (less than 3.5 hours per week) accounted for 31 percent of all premature deaths among the study participants, with 59 percent of the deaths attributable to cardiovascular disease and 21 percent from cancer among the non-smoking women. The researchers concluded: "It is clear that both weight and exercise are important for health and longevity. There is no question that you should be as active as possible no matter what your weight is, but it is equally important to maintain a healthy weight and prevent weight gain through diet and lifestyle."

We can't afford to ignore the health consequences of obesity. We need to take steps now to adopt a healthier lifestyle. Keep in mind that even small losses lead to great health rewards. Studies show that if you are overweight, losing even 5–10 percent of that excess weight can dramatically improve your health by lowering your blood pressure, cholesterol levels, and blood sugar. Plus, you will have more energy, sleep better, and enjoy better overall health.

By now you should have a more thorough understanding of obesity and the factors that contribute to weight gain. To reach and maintain a healthy weight, you need to learn to make critical distinctions between weight loss and fat loss, between diet and nutrition, and between being thin and being healthy. Let's now take an in-depth look at the glycemic index and how and why balancing blood sugar is so valuable to weight loss and reducing your risk of developing chronic diseases.

2
WHAT IS THE GLYCEMIC INDEX?

$\mathcal{T}$he glycemic index (GI) is a tool that can help people lose weight and assist in the prevention and management of diabetes and heart disease. The GI is a ranking of carbohydrates based on how quickly they are broken down and how they affect blood sugar. Also called blood glucose, blood sugar is the fuel that the body's cells use for energy. Carbohydrates that are digested rapidly and broken down quickly into blood glucose are ranked as high GI. These include refined starches such as processed breakfast cereals (corn flakes) and white bread and bagels. Carbohydrates that are more slowly digested and broken down into blood glucose have a low GI. Examples include most vegetables, non-tropical fruits, and unprocessed grains. Low-GI foods have a less dramatic impact on blood sugar and help keep levels more balanced.

Eating high-GI foods can lead to blood sugar highs and lows, which may result in fatigue, increased appetite, and food cravings, particularly for sweets. Also, numerous studies have linked diets that include large amounts of high-GI foods to obesity, increased belly fat, insulin resistance, type 2 diabetes, high cholesterol, and increased risk factors for heart disease. On the other hand, research indicates that choosing carbohydrates that are low GI as well as healthy can help bring about weight loss and reduce body fat, especially around the abdomen. Having good blood sugar balance can also promote a more even mood, reduce hunger cravings, and increase metabolic rate, which are all important factors in promoting long-term weight management and preventing chronic diseases. For all of these reasons, it is best to minimize your intake of high-GI foods and maximize your intake of low-GI foods. This book can show you how.

A New View on Carbohydrates

The term "glycemic index" was first coined by professors David Jenkins and Tom Wolever from the Department of Nutritional Sciences, Faculty of Medicine, University of Toronto in Canada. Their research paper "Glycemic Index of Foods: A Physiological Basis for Carbohydrate Exchange" was published in 1981 in the *American Journal of Clinical Nutrition* and revolutionized the way people understood the role of carbohydrates in the diet. The researchers wanted to take an in-depth look at the food recommendations for diabetics. At that time carbohydrates were classified as either simple (sugars) or complex (starches and vegetables). It was believed that all simple carbohydrates caused a rapid rise in blood glucose levels and all complex carbohydrates released glucose more slowly into the body. Consequently, diabetics were advised to limit intake of simple carbohydrates and eat more complex carbohydrates to manage their blood sugar.

After the Canadian research was published, however, a whole new view of carbohydrates emerged that challenged this previously held belief. Jenkins and Wolever's results showed that the glycemic (blood glucose) response of carbohydrates was not black and white; in fact, blood glucose responses varied considerably among various complex carbohydrates. The researchers concluded that certain carbohydrates were of better quality than others. The biggest surprise was that certain starchy foods (such as white bread) were digested and absorbed more quickly than certain sugary foods. These results went against what was believed at the time. As a result, the research paper fueled a dramatic increase in curiosity, debate, and ultimately clinical research on this topic all around the world. Nutrition and medical experts, especially those working with people with diabetes, obesity, and heart disease, started to re-examine their recommendations for carbohydrate and sugar intake. Instead of only describing carbohydrates as complex or simple, now carbohydrates were also defined as low or high GI, and dietary recommendations were made accordingly.

How Is the Glycemic Index Measured?

The GI is a system of ranking all forms of carbohydrates (breads, rice, pasta, legumes, fruits, and vegetables) on a scale of zero to 100 according to their glycemic response, which is how a carbohydrate affects blood glucose levels and consequently insulin levels (insulin is the hormone released by the pancreas to take glucose from the bloodstream and escort it to cells for energy utilization or storage as fat). In the GI scale, zero is the equivalent of water, which does not have any impact on blood glucose levels, and 100 is the equivalent of pure glucose (sugar).

If a food is digested quickly, causing a rapid rise in blood glucose, it is categorized as a high-GI food. Examples include white bread and bagels, soda crackers, and baked potatoes. When you eat high-GI foods, there is a quick increase in blood sugar, providing what is known as the *sugar high* or *sugar rush*. At this point you feel energized; however, the feeling does not last. In response to this rapid rise in blood sugar, the pancreas will overproduce insulin, which results in a subsequent fall in blood sugar. So, while high-GI foods can be counted on to provide us with bursts of energy, this energy is not sustainable and is followed by an equally dramatic drop in energy (or *sugar low*) that may cause feelings of fatigue, sluggishness, slowed mental function, increased hunger and cravings, and sudden irritability. To counter these sugar lows, people crave and then consume more high-GI foods, only to start the vicious bingeing-craving cycle all over again. Plus, as you will read about in the next chapter, insulin highs can promote fat storage, along with a lot of other problems.

Carbohydrates that are digested more slowly, causing a gradual release of blood glucose into the body, are categorized as a low GI.

Examples include pumpernickel bread, chickpeas, green vegetables, apples, and oat bran. These foods provide the body with sustained energy, which reduces hunger and improves the manner in which the body uses energy reserves (stored fat).

This graph below illustrates how low- versus high-GI foods affect our blood glucose levels. As you can see, there is a dramatic rise and fall in blood sugar that occurs when high-GI foods are eaten. Continually eating these foods throughout the day (riding the sugar rollercoaster) can have a significant impact on your energy levels, cognitive function, appetite, and ability to burn fat.

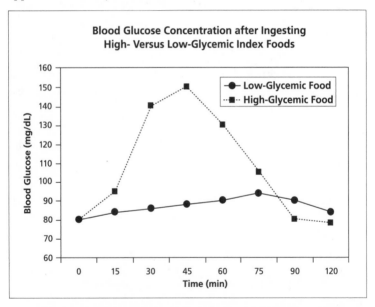

To date, more than 700 foods have been classified according to their glycemic index. The GI value of a food is determined using scientific methods and cannot be calculated by simply analyzing the composition of a food. Currently, only a few nutrition research groups around the world provide a legitimate testing service. For over a decade, Professor Jennie Brand-Miller, of the Human Nutrition Unit at the University of Sydney, Australia, and co-author of *The New Glucose Revolution* and *The Low GI Diet Revolution*, has been at the forefront of glycemic index research. This research unit has measured the GI values of more than 400 foods and counting. There is a GI value chart in Chapter 7. For a more comprehensive list, go to: www.glycemicindex.com

Brand-Miller and her colleagues obtain a GI rating by feeding a portion of a food containing 50 grams of carbohydrate to 10 healthy study participants who have fasted overnight. Blood samples are taken at 15- to 30-minute intervals for two hours afterward. At another time, the same 10 people eat an equal carbohydrate portion of glucose sugar (referred to as the reference food) and again have their blood glucose responses measured for two hours. The results from these tests are plotted on a graph. The area under each curve (AUC) is calculated to reflect the participants total rise in blood glucose levels after they have eaten the test and reference foods. The GI rating is calculated by dividing the AUC for the test food by the AUC for the control food, and multiplying the result by100. The average of the GI ratings from all 10 participants is considered to be the official GI of that food.

Here are the reference ranges for the glycemic index:
Low GI = 55 or less
Moderate GI = 56–69
High GI = 70 or higher

Factors That Influence the Glycemic Index

GI values reflect the average glucose response when a particular carbohydrate is eaten and not combined with any other foods. The values are also measured after a night of fasting, so that the results are not affected by anything else in the stomach. In real life, we eat carbohydrates along with other foods that can impact the glycemic response of the meal. Fat and protein will cause carbohydrates to be digested more slowly, thus changing the overall glycemic impact of a meal. For example, eating chicken and almonds along with rice will have a lower glycemic impact than eating just the rice alone. There are a variety of other factors that influence the glycemic index of a food, such as:

- *The type of sugar:* Fructose, which is found in many fruits, some vegetables, and honey, is broken down more slowly in the body compared to sucrose (table sugar). This explains in part why fruit, which is sweet, is lower in the GI compared to other sweets (jelly beans). Fruit also contains soluble fiber, which lowers the GI.

- *The type of starch:* Amylose starch, which is found in basmati rice, contains glucose rings that are hooked together, making it harder to digest, so foods containing this starch will have a lower GI rank. Amylopectin starch is easier to digest, so foods containing this starch have a higher GI value (for example, jasmine rice).

- *Acid content of the food:* Acid slows down the digestion of a food. For example, adding balsamic vinegar to your meals can reduce the glycemic response. Sourdough bread, which is made by slow fermentation of flour by yeasts, contains more organic acids, resulting in a much lower GI compared to white bread.

- *Fiber content:* The more soluble fiber there is in a carbohydrate, the lower the GI. Soluble fiber swells with water and causes the food to break down more slowly into sugar. This is why whole grains, which contain more soluble fiber, are lower GI.

- *Cooking:* Heating can increase the GI ranking of a food. Cooking swells the starch molecules, making them quicker to digest. For example, raw carrots have a lower GI than cooked carrots. Cooking pasta *al dente* gives it a lower GI rating compared to cooking it to a soft consistency.

- *Processing of a food:* Highly processed and refined foods are usually digested quickly and have a higher GI. For example, refining whole wheat into white flour will result in a higher GI of foods made with that flour. The same is true of rice—white rice has a higher GI than brown rice.

What Is the Glycemic Load?

Now that you have a better understanding of the glycemic index, we can look at another term—the "glycemic load." The glycemic load was created by researchers at Harvard University to help us understand how a specific serving size of a carbohydrate food will impact blood sugar. It takes into consideration both the glycemic index and the grams of carbohydrate in a particular serving. Recall that when the GI is calculated, researchers use a portion size of a food that provides 50 grams of carbohydrate to allow for standardized testing. The 50 grams is not the serving size, but the amount of carbohydrate in the food. For example, watermelon is rated high GI; however, it takes 5 cups of watermelon to provide 50 grams of carbohydrate. If you eat a smaller portion of watermelon it will not have as great an impact on your blood sugar. There are many other fruits and vegetables that are listed moderate to high in the GI but because they contain a small amount of carbohydrate per serving, their overall impact on blood glucose levels is not that great. In reality we don't eat these "standardized" amounts of food. We eat varied portions, so in order to figure out how our particular portion of food will impact our blood sugar we can use the glycemic load.

Here is how the glycemic load is calculated:
Step 1: Start with the glycemic index rating of a single carbohydrate food and multiply that number by the amount (grams) of carbohydrate in the particular portion (this is available on label packaging or at www. glycemicindex.com).
Step 2: Take that resulting number and divide it by100.

Here is an example:
The glycemic index for mango is 60 (moderate). There are 15.1 grams of carbohydrate in a 120-gram serving. The glycemic load is (60 × 15.1) ÷ 100 = 9.1 (low).

This is a perfect example of a food that has a high glycemic index but a low glycemic load because it contains a small amount of carbohydrates in a typical serving. Again, keep in mind that even if a food is moderate or high GI, if it contains very few carbohydrates per serving (such as watermelon, mango, and other fruits and vegetables), then the impact on blood sugar and insulin levels will not be great. If a food has both a high GI ranking and a high carbohydrate content (such as white bread, potatoes, and white rice), it will have a high glycemic load and should be eaten in limited amounts.

Here are the reference ranges for the glycemic load:
Low glycemic load = 10 or less
Moderate glycemic load = 11–19
High glycemic load = 20 and higher

Using the GI and GL for Meal Planning

It is not necessary to memorize the GI ratings of foods or do GL calculations for every carbohydrate you eat. Simply familiarize yourself with the GI chart in Chapter 7 (make a copy and post it on your fridge). Use the GL when you want to know how much of a particular food you should eat. You will find both GI and GL values at www.glycemicindex.com. In general, low-GI foods can be eaten in larger portions while high-GI foods should be eaten in smaller portions to manage glycemic load. *That doesn't mean that you can eat low-GI foods in unlimited amounts. It is important to keep the total glycemic load low at each meal.* When the total glycemic load of a meal is high, it triggers hormonal changes that promote fat storage. When the total glycemic load of a meal is low, it triggers your body to start actively using fat as an energy source.

For example, spaghetti is 45 on the GI, which is moderate, but you shouldn't eat massive portions. One cup or about 180 grams of white spaghetti contains about 44.8 grams of carbohydrate. This translates into 20.2 on the GL, which is high, but still okay in moderation. However, if you have two or three 1-cup helpings, that can be a problem. If you combine your 1 cup of pasta with 2 cups of a sauce that contains vegetables (low GI), you will have a satisfying meal that is easy on your blood sugar.

Lastly, remember that you can't go wrong with fruits and vegetables, even if they are moderate to high GI, because they contain smaller amounts of carbohydrates and are excellent sources of vitamins, minerals, and fiber.

So, Is the GI the Next "It" Diet?

Don't misinterpret the hype surrounding the glycemic index. Although following a low-GI diet can help promote weight loss, you will achieve the best results if you combine a low-GI diet with regular exercise, adequate sleep, stress management, and smart supplements.

Following a low-GI diet is not a fad; this is a new way of eating that is here to stay and that's what makes it so important. It's a revolutionary way of understanding and choosing foods, and here's why: This sensible approach to eating is metabolism-driven, promotes satiety (satisfaction from meals), allows for variances in the diet, and has significant, well-documented benefits for overall health.

The chart of low/moderate/high-GI carbohydrate values (which appears on page 89 of this book) offers you a guide when choosing which carbohydrates to consume. Eating low-GI foods is healthy, nutritious, and easy to follow. This is particularly important because most fad diets, such as the low-carb or no-carb diets, are difficult to sustain over the long term, and can be detrimental to your health. The GI offers an alternative that allows the intake of carbohydrates, but promotes the consumption of low-GI carbohydrates such as fruits, vegetables, whole grains, legumes, and nuts, which are the healthy, high-fiber carbohydrates. More importantly, the GI offers significant benefits for controlling blood sugar and lowering the risk of chronic diseases.

The Health Benefits of Eating Low-GI Foods

The health benefits of a low-GI diet are widespread and well documented. They include improved weight control, enhanced blood sugar management, and, most importantly, decreased risk of diabetes, high cholesterol, and heart disease. Over time, a low-GI diet can promote fat loss, especially around the abdomen, and modify appetite and food cravings to a more normal level. Digestion and bowel function can improve since eating more vegetables, fruit, and other quality sources of soluble fiber can lessen constipation and diarrhea. Finally, there are secondary benefits to having better blood sugar control, such as more energy and vitality, a better mood, and improved sleep patterns. I have provided a summary of some of the key research on the glycemic index at the back of this book.

All of the benefits from a low-GI diet begin and end with enhanced blood sugar and insulin management. Let's take a closer look at this topic to better understand the role of insulin in your health.

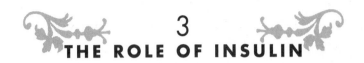

3
THE ROLE OF INSULIN

*I*nsulin is often thought of only in its relationship to people with diabetes, yet insulin plays a vital role in the functioning of every cell in the body. Furthermore, insulin is one of the hormones critical in fat storage, so if you are interested in losing weight or preventing weight gain, then it is important to understand the role of insulin.

When we eat carbohydrates, they are broken down during digestion into glucose. As glucose enters the blood, it causes a rise in blood sugar. The pancreas responds by releasing insulin, which transports sugar from the bloodstream into the cells throughout the body, where it can be utilized as energy, so insulin helps return blood sugar levels to normal. Insulin also aids in the production of enzymes, hormones, and muscle.

Understanding Insulin Resistance

When blood sugar levels are balanced, the body functions in its optimal state. Throughout the day, blood sugar levels naturally fluctuate, meaning blood sugar levels rise modestly after a meal, insulin is released to bring blood sugar into the cells to be used for energy, and then blood sugar levels return to normal. However, if we eat too many refined, high-glycemic carbohydrates, insulin levels must increase to bring the body back to balance. If insulin levels are chronically elevated, then the cells of your body can eventually become resistant to the action of insulin. This condition is called *insulin resistance* and once it occurs, insulin becomes ineffective in moving glucose into the cells to be burned for energy, so blood glucose levels remain high. This scenario is the precursor to type 2 diabetes. It is estimated that over 25 percent of the population suffer with high blood glucose levels and insulin resistance.

A high-GI diet has been shown to increase the risk of developing insulin resistance. Other factors that can increase risk include:

- *Genetics:* Inherited defects with insulin receptors

- *Inactivity:* Lack of exercise reduces the muscles' sensitivity to insulin

- *Obesity:* Body fat releases a hormone called resistin, which reduces insulin sensitivity

Insulin Resistance: A Slippery Slope to Illness

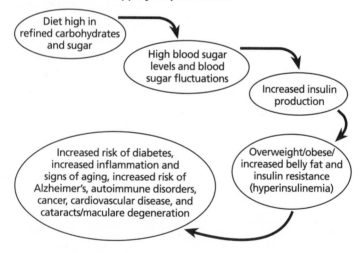

Insulin resistance occurs when the body becomes resistant or "immune" to the action of its own insulin. In addition to being a known risk factor for type 2 diabetes, insulin resistance is associated with increased risk of obesity, cardiovascular disease, kidney disease, nerve damage, and polycystic ovarian syndrome.

Insulin, Prediabetes, and Diabetes

If you have insulin resistance, your cells (muscle, fat, and liver cells) do not use insulin properly, so blood sugar levels remain high. In response, the pancreas releases more insulin to try and reduce blood glucose levels. The end result is high, uncontrolled blood glucose *and* high insulin levels, known as hyperglycemia and hyperinsulinemia, respectively.

People with blood glucose levels that are higher than normal but not yet in the diabetic range have prediabetes. This is also referred to as impaired glucose tolerance. Prediabetes is becoming a widespread problem in North America. According to some estimates, over 54 million American adults had prediabetes in 2002, and those numbers were expected to rise.

In the prediabetic stage, the pancreas works hard to keep up with the added demand by producing more insulin. Over time, though, insulin secretion from the pancreas falters, and the pancreas cannot secrete enough insulin in response to meals, leading to full-blown type 2 diabetes, which accounts for approximately 90 percent of all diabetes cases. In the past, this form was called adult-onset or non-insulin dependent diabetes. The greatest increase of type 2 diabetes in recent years has occurred among children and adolescents.

This progression from insulin resistance to prediabetes to diabetes doesn't happen overnight. Studies have shown that most people with insulin resistance and prediabetes go on to develop type 2 diabetes within 10 years, so there is a long period of "warning." The problem is that often there are no initial symptoms of insulin resistance and prediabetes. You may have one or both conditions for several years without noticing anything. If you have a severe form of insulin resistance, you may get dark patches of skin on the back of your neck, elbows, knees, or knuckles. This condition is called *acanthosis nigricans*. Once diabetes occurs, there may be symptoms of mood swings, irritability, hunger, thirst, and food cravings.

Blood Sugar Highs and Lows

Insulin is critical in the transportation and processing of glucose into usable energy, and a lack of it results in increased blood glucose levels, a condition known as hyperglycemia. Symptoms of hyperglycemia include excessive thirst, hunger, and urination. Chronic hyperglycemia can cause dry mouth, itchy skin, fatigue, and recurrent infections. Hypoglycemia, on the other hand, occurs when blood sugar levels drop below normal levels, causing dizziness, shaking, sudden sweating and nausea, a racing heart, and general mental confusion. The symptoms may be temporary until blood sugar levels are restored. Hypoglycemia may occur for those with diabetes, but may also be triggered by poor diet and lifestyle. Both hyper- and hypoglycemia may be precursors to diabetes and can have serious, even fatal consequences if left untreated. If you suffer the symptoms of either condition, consult your health care provider immediately to determine the root cause, and to address diet and lifestyle factors.

Blood tests can be used to determine if you have prediabetes or diabetes. A fasting blood glucose test measures your blood sugar level after an overnight fast. Type 2 diabetes is defined as a fasting plasma glucose level of 126 mg/dL (7.0 mmol/L) or higher. Another test, called the glucose tolerance test, is done secondary to the fasting blood glucose test. This test measures blood glucose levels two hours after you've drunk a glucose solution. A reading of greater than 198 mg/dL (11 mmol/L) indicates diabetes.

These tests, along with fasting insulin tests, are helpful in determining whether a person has insulin resistance. Anyone over age 45 who is also overweight or obese should have these tests done. Other risk factors for type 2 diabetes include: a family history of diabetes, poor diet (high intake of refined starches and sugars—high-GI foods), an inactive lifestyle, high blood pressure or cholesterol, and ethnicity (Black, Hispanic, and Native Americans are at higher risk).

Deadly Connection

The link between obesity, insulin resistance, and type 2 diabetes is very strong. Over 80 percent of people with type 2 diabetes are overweight or obese and 92 percent of people with type 2 diabetes have insulin resistance. Studies have shown that losing 5–7 percent of body weight, through changes in diet and activity level, can prevent the progression from insulin resistance to diabetes.

The other main form of diabetes is called type 1 diabetes, which was previously known as juvenile-onset diabetes because it occurs primarily in children or adolescents. This form accounts for only about 10 percent of diabetes cases. In type 1 diabetes, the cells that produce insulin (beta cells) become damaged or are destroyed and can no longer produce enough insulin to manage blood sugar. In infants and children, beta cells are usually destroyed rapidly, causing a sudden rise in blood sugar levels. In adults, they are destroyed more slowly, causing a slower rise in blood sugar levels. Typically, people with type 1 diabetes need to have insulin injections to control their blood sugar levels. Insulin resistance can also occur in people who have type 1 diabetes, especially if they are overweight.

International Diabetes Statistics

In 1998, the World Health Organization published a report that estimated the number of people with diabetes was 135 million worldwide. However, less than a decade later, that estimate jumped to 194 million. According to the International Diabetes Federation, diabetes now affects more than 230 million people worldwide and is expected to affect 350 million by 2025. Diabetes is the fourth or fifth leading cause of death in developed countries, and is responsible for over one million amputations each year. In 2003, the countries with the highest population of diabetics were India (35.5 million), China (23.8 million), the United States (16 million), Russia (9.7 million), and Japan (6.7 million). By 2025, the number of people with diabetes is expected to more than double in Africa, the Eastern Mediterranean, the Middle East, and Southeast Asia. The incidence of diabetes is expected to rise by 20 percent in Europe, 50 percent in North America, 85 percent in South and Central America, and 75 percent in the Western Pacific.

Insulin and Metabolic Syndrome: What's the Connection?

Metabolic syndrome, formerly called Syndrome X, is a term given to a collection of symptoms that increase one's risk of heart disease, stroke, and diabetes. The underlying cause of metabolic syndrome is insulin resistance. It is the key factor to creating the metabolic changes that lead to weight gain, elevated cholesterol, high blood pressure, and then eventually type 2 diabetes and heart disease. Each of these factors alone is dangerous to health, but having them together greatly increases the risk of developing chronic diseases.

Metabolic syndrome is diagnosed when a person has three or more of the following characteristics:

- Abdominal obesity—waist circumference greater than 40 inches (102 cm) in men, and 35 inches (89 cm) in women
- High triglyceride levels—above 150 mg/dL (1.7 mmol/L)
- Low HDL cholesterol levels—less than 40 mg/dL (1 mmol/L) in men, and 50 mg/dL (1.3 mmol/L) in women
- High blood pressure—greater than or equal to 130/85 mm Hg
- Insulin resistance
- High fasting glucose level—with fasting blood sugar more than 110 mg/dL (6.2 mmol/L)

Some experts estimate that as many as one in four, or 47 million adults in the United States, have metabolic syndrome. These numbers are expected to increase as the population ages. Age is not the cause of metabolic syndrome; however, the key risk factors for developing this condition—inactivity and obesity—are simply more prevalent in older adults. In fact, approximately 40 percent of those over age 60 have metabolic syndrome.

Insulin and Appetite: What's the Connection?

Insulin has widespread influence on the body, and affects digestion, metabolism, and appetite. Studies show that regular consumption of high-glycemic meals can increase appetite and cravings for carbohydrates. High-GI foods are digested quickly, causing a rapid rise in blood sugar—at this point, you feel good. However, once insulin is released, your blood sugar levels start to drop off, making you feel tired, moody, and hungry. So the energy burst is temporary and followed by a crash, which prompts us to snack on more high-glycemic foods.

Conversely, low-GI foods, such as vegetables, fruits, and whole grains, are digested and absorbed more slowly, providing a sustained release of energy and a longer feeling of fullness from a meal. By preventing blood sugar highs and lows, a low-GI diet can help to control cravings and appetite. This slow release of glucose into the bloodstream means that after-meal insulin levels are lowered, which helps to maintain insulin sensitivity. Plus, these foods generally provide rich sources of vitamins, minerals, and fiber, which are essential nutrients for good health.

Insulin and Body Fat: What's the Connection?

Insulin resistance and body fat share a reciprocal and rather unhealthy relationship. High insulin levels cause us to store more fat, and carrying excess fat increases the risk of insulin resistance. Does this sound confusing? Let me explain.

Insulin is intimately connected to our potential for fat burning and fat storage. High insulin levels reduce the levels of lipoprotein lipase, the enzyme that releases fat from storage to be used as energy. As a result, more fat is stored because that enzyme is reduced. On the flip side, low insulin levels increase a hormone called glucagon, which allows fat to be burned for energy. As long as insulin levels remain high, fat remains in storage and the body will continue to use glucose for its energy needs.

To burn fat for energy and to reduce belly fat, blood sugar levels must be balanced and insulin levels must be lowered. This can be achieved through proper diet, nutritional supplements, and exercise, as outlined in the coming chapters.

Insulin, Stress, and Cortisol: What's the Connection?

Cortisol is a hormone released from the adrenal glands in response to stress or those "fight or flight" situations (rush hour traffic, deadlines). Approximately half of all adults suffer the adverse effects of stress, such as muscle tension, high blood pressure, insomnia, and depression. Most recently, stress has been linked to obesity. When a person experiences chronic stress, cortisol levels rise. This causes the body to store more fat around the belly, which reduces insulin sensitivity.

The news on cortisol is not all bad. Cortisol is the most important hormone for blood sugar and insulin regulation. In response to a stressful event, cortisol helps your body become more effective at producing glucose from protein, a process called gluconeogenesis, so that it can accommodate the increased energy requirements. This protein comes from existing body structures, such as muscle, skin, and organs. It is not a problem if this happens only occasionally and is short term. However, when stress is chronic, this process can lead to muscle loss (wasting), another factor that can contribute to weight gain because loss of muscle means that metabolism is reduced.

During stress, cortisol reduces insulin sensitivity and the utilization of glucose for energy so that there is increased blood sugar available to be used by the central nervous system or your brain. Your brain is the only organ in the body that can absorb glucose directly without the action of insulin. Your brain uses approximately 100 grams of glucose daily, and during times of high stress, it demands even more. Cortisol increases the amount of glucose available to accommodate the brain's increased desire for glucose. Researchers believe that insulin resistance develops in part as a coping mechanism to feed the brain with necessary glucose.

The release of cortisol in response to stress was designed to help the body quickly increase energy supplies to meet the immediate demands. However, because chronic stress levels associated with Western lifestyles keep us in this "fight or flight" mode continuously, the risk of developing full-blown insulin resistance increases (from a prolonged decrease in insulin sensitivity) and weight gain occurs (remember, excess insulin increases fat storage).

Stress isn't the only factor that raises cortisol. Eating too many sweet, simple carbohydrates can also elevate cortisol levels. When you eat a high-GI food, such as a jelly beans, the body generates a strong insulin response to reduce blood sugar. This strong insulin response can trigger a dramatic drop in blood sugar for three to five hours after the snack. When blood glucose levels fall, this triggers a surge of adrenaline and cortisol. This can result in anxiety, irritability, nervousness, and palpitations. Continual consumption of high-GI, sugary foods can lead to fluctuations of insulin, glucose, and adrenal hormones throughout the day, with consequences on both physical and emotional well-being.

Insulin and Aging: What's the Connection?

Poorly regulated blood sugar and insulin levels are major contributors to accelerated aging. As production and effectiveness of insulin falters, glucose builds up in the bloodstream, causing a series of health problems that many people associate with normal aging. For example, we have all heard the expression 'midlife spread.' Gaining fat around the abdomen is a consequence of uncontrolled blood sugar, insulin resistance, stress, and lack of activity. People mistakenly think that weight gain is a result of aging when in reality it is a sign of an underlying hormonal imbalance and of course lifestyle factors.

Excess blood sugar can bind to proteins in skin, cartilage, muscle, blood vessels, and other tissues, causing wrinkling, stiffening, and malfunctioning, leading to accelerated aging. When blood vessels and nerves become stiff and hardened, blood flow to the organs and extremities is impaired. In the extremities this can feel like pins and needles or numbness in the hands and feet. Poor circulation to the blood vessels in the pelvic area can result in erectile dysfunction, which is discussed in more detail below.

If hemoglobin (the oxygen-binding protein in red blood cells) is encrusted with glucose, then the brain, heart, and muscles receive less oxygen, causing all functions to decrease. This results in lack of energy and premature aging. Connective tissue (collagen) is also affected by excess sugar, resulting in skin wrinkles. Cataracts may develop as a result of damage to the lens of the eye, which is made of protein. If the same problem affects the retina, blindness may occur. Mental acuity may also be affected.

Insulin also activates genes that encourage inflammation, so with high insulin, the level of inflammation in your body increases. Joints become swollen and inflexible as the symptoms of arthritis set in.

High blood sugar and elevated insulin may increase your risk of degenerative brain diseases such as dementia and Alzheimer's disease. But that's not all—high blood glucose levels affect the function of many proteins and enzymes, so that the chances of dying prematurely *from any cause* are higher. You don't need to be in the diabetic range to be at risk. High glucose and insulin levels fuel the growth of abnormal cells that cause various types of cancer, including breast, colon, endometrial, and pancreatic.

Insulin and Heart Disease: What's the Connection?

Heart disease claims more lives every year than any other affliction, and is particularly worrisome for diabetics. According to the American Heart Association, 63 percent of people with diabetes experience symptoms of cardiovascular disease. In fact, the AHA estimates that three-quarters of people with diabetes will die of some form of heart or blood vessel disease.

It is not just diabetics who need to be worried about heart disease. Those with prediabetes and those who eat high-glycemic diets are also at increased risk of heart disease for a variety of reasons. Uncontrolled high blood glucose levels can cause damage to the blood vessels of the heart. Having high insulin levels (hyperinsulinemia) and insulin resistance is associated with obesity, hypertension, hyperlipidemia (elevated cholesterol), and diabetes—all major risk factors for heart disease. As well, a study published in the *American Journal of Clinical Nutrition* in 2002 reported a significant association between diets with a high glycemic load and increased levels of C-reactive protein (a protein indicator of inflammation and a distinct marker for disease, particularly heart disease).

Obesity itself is a major risk factor for heart disease. Excess body weight increases the workload and stress to the heart, which causes blood pressure to rise. When insulin levels are high, the body retains sodium, which also increases blood pressure.

The connection between insulin and cholesterol is a little more complicated. High insulin levels trigger the release of free fatty acids into the bloodstream. The liver responds by increasing triglycerides, which increase high-density lipoprotein (HDL) excretion from the body, lowering your blood HDL (good) cholesterol levels. These changes also cause the LDL (bad) cholesterol to become smaller and more dense, which makes it more likely to form as plaque on the inside of blood vessels. So, to summarize, the net result of high insulin is elevated triglycerides, low HDL cholesterol, and an increase in small, dense LDL cholesterol, a combination of factors known to substantially increase the risk of cardiovascular disease.

The good news is that studies show that following a diet of low-GI foods improves insulin response and can reduce risk factors for heart disease. Specifically, a low-GI diet has been shown to increase levels of HDL cholesterol and decrease levels of LDL cholesterol. Several reports also indicate that low-glycemic diets are associated with lower triglyceride levels (a marker for heart health). One study published in the *Current Atherosclerosis Reports* (Nov. 3, 2001) found that substituting low-GI for high-GI foods can lower triglycerides by 15–25 percent. A low-GI diet can also help facilitate weight loss, which in turn helps reduce two other risk factors for heart disease: high blood pressure and high cholesterol.

Heart Disease Wake-up Call!

According to the Center for Disease Control in the US, cardiovascular disease (CVD) is the leading cause of death in men and women in Canada, the US, China, Europe, and Australia. Heart attack and stroke are responsible for twice as many deaths in women in the US than are all forms of cancer combined. Both the World Heart Organization and the World Health Organization report that CVD kills up to 17 million people each year. In developing countries, CVD is on the rise, afflicting people at an earlier age than in developed nations. Up to 80 percent of the world's deaths by CVD are now reported in developing or middle-income nations. By 2020, CVD will be the leading cause of death worldwide (with the exception of sub-Saharan Africa), surpassing communicable diseases. However, there is hope. National education efforts and individual action can reduce the risk of disability or death from CVD by up to 50 percent. The leading risk factors for CVD include, in order, hypertension, high blood cholesterol, diabetes, obesity, cigarette smoking, and inactivity. These are what we call modifiable risk factors because we have control over them.

Insulin, Blood Sugar, and Sexual Function

One of the less commonly talked about or known implications of poor blood sugar control and insulin resistance is erectile dysfunction (ED), the inability to get or maintain an erection. Essentially, ED occurs when there is a breakdown in the sequence of events that normally lead to an erection. This disruption can occur in nerve impulses to and from the brain, spine, and penis, or in the muscles, fibrous tissues, and arteries in or near the corpora cavernosa (the two parallel chambers of the penis that fill with blood to create an erection).

Excess insulin in the bloodstream created by insulin resistance can damage the endothelium of the blood vessels (the layer on the inside of blood vessels that secretes chemicals which instruct the vessel to contract or relax). To achieve an erection, a substance called nitric oxide must be released from the endothelium to allow the blood vessels to dilate and fill with blood. If the endothelium is damaged by excess insulin and releases less nitric oxide to the penis, it will lessen or prevent the blood vessels from dilating and can lead to ED. It is estimated that about 35–50 percent of men with diabetes experience ED. Those with insulin resistance and prediabetes are also at increased risk due to elevated blood sugar levels, which damage the blood vessels.

Now that you have a good understanding of the role of insulin and the consequences of uncontrolled blood sugar and insulin resistance, let's take a look at the nutritional strategies and principles that are key for following a low-glycemic diet.

4
MACRONUTRIENTS

*F*ollowing a low-GI diet involves using the glycemic index as a tool for making healthy carbohydrate choices. While the GI is valuable, there are other dietary factors to consider. In order to lose weight and prevent chronic diseases, it is also important to make smart choices with fats and protein.

Together, carbohydrates, protein, and fats are called macronutrients because we need them in large quantities ("macro"), compared to the micronutrients (vitamins and minerals), which are needed in smaller quantities. We need a balance of high-quality protein, carbohydrates, and fats in order to function at our best. These macronutrients provide us with the energy and building blocks required for proper growth, development, and many body processes.

Numerous fad diets over the years have focused on cutting carbs or fats, yet these approaches were not successful and came at a price. Not getting enough quality carbohydrates can cause fatigue, depression, and nutrient deficiencies, and a lack of essential fats can cause skin and hair problems, inflammation, depression, and other health concerns. We also need to be careful not to get excessive amounts of these foods (especially high-GI carbs, saturated fats, and trans fats) as that can result in weight gain and increased risk of heart disease, diabetes, and other problems. There are good and bad types of macronutrients; striking the right balance is the key to optimal health and weight management. In this chapter I will sort through the myths and misconceptions about macronutrients and give you advice on how to make the best choices.

Recommended Macronutrient Intake

The US Institute of Medicine recommends ranges for macronutrient intake that are associated with a reduced risk of chronic diseases while providing adequate intake of essential nutrients. It suggests that adults get 45–65 percent of their calories from carbohydrates, 20–35 percent from fat, and 10–35 percent from protein. Ranges for children are similar, except that infants and younger children need a slightly higher proportion of fat (25–40 percent).

Carbohydrates: Cutting Through the Confusion

We have discussed carbohydrates and their relationship to blood sugar and insulin, but there is more to know about this heavily scrutinized food group.

Carbohydrates are the body's main source of fuel, glucose, which is needed by every cell in our bodies. They also provide valuable nutrients (vitamins, minerals, and essential fatty acids) and fiber, which is important for many aspects of health.

Carbohydrates are found in cereals and grains, legumes, vegetables, fruits, and dairy products. In the past they were classified as either simple or complex and we were told to limit intake of simple carbohydrates (sugars) and eat more complex carbohydrates (starches and grains). However, we now know that complex carbohydrates vary greatly in quality and how they are processed in the body. Some complex carbohydrates (such as white bread and jasmine rice) are processed more quickly into sugar than simple carbohydrates. Thus the glycemic index is now the preferred way of classifying carbohydrates. As discussed earlier, choosing primarily low- and moderate-GI carbohydrates can help improve blood glucose control and support weight loss.

The Fiber Factor

Dietary fiber is found in fruits, vegetables, beans, and the indigestible parts of whole grains such as wheat and oat bran. In addition to supporting intestinal health and proper elimination, fiber improves blood sugar balance, lowers cholesterol, reduces the risk of colon and breast cancer, and plays a role in weight management.

There are two types of dietary fiber: insoluble and soluble. Both forms are found in most foods, but in varying amounts. Foods that contain good amounts of insoluble fiber include beans and lentils, brown rice, fruits with edible seeds, celery, green beans, oats, flaxseed, and wheat and corn bran. Insoluble fiber has a bulking effect in the stomach, which slows digestion and absorption. It also improves elimination (and relieves constipation) by absorbing water and swelling within the intestine, which helps pull and remove waste materials from the body.

Soluble fiber can be found in all fruit and vegetables in varying amounts. Good sources include legumes, oats, rye, psyllium seed husk, root vegetables (potatoes and carrots), plums, apples, and strawberries. Soluble fiber mixes with water in a meal to form a gel in the stomach, which traps waste and helps lower LDL (bad) cholesterol. It also slows down the rate of digestion and lowers a food's GI.

The recommended daily intake of fiber for adults 50 years and younger is 38 grams for men and 25 grams for women; for men and women over 50 the recommended intake is 30 and 21 grams per day, respectively, due to decreased food consumption. Most people get only half of the recommended amount of fiber. To boost your intake, incorporate more raw vegetables, fruits, and legumes in your diet. Choose whole grains (brown bread/rice/pasta and whole oats) over refined products as the refining process strips away most of the fiber and nutrients. These foods are also lower in the GI and highly nutritious. If you are not getting enough fiber in your diet, consider taking a supplement. Look for a product that contains a blend of soluble and insoluble fibers. When increasing your fiber intake, do so gradually to minimize the possibility of gas or bloating that may otherwise occur.

Sugar: Not So Sweet

Sweets are a weakness for many of us and sugar has become far too prevalent in our diet. According to Statistics Canada, the average Canadian consumes 23 teaspoons of added sugar every day. This translates into approximately 92 pounds of sugar per year. And this figure includes only refined sugars, honey, and maple syrup, not the added sugars we get from corn sweeteners (the main ingredient in pop) or the sugars in fruit juices. According to US Department of Agriculture data, the average teenage boy eats at least 109 pounds per year. This is not surprising when you consider the amount of soda pop, candy, and junk food that teenagers are eating today.

The obvious sources of sugar are soda pop, candy, cookies, and other baked goods, but most of us don't think about the hidden sources, such as ketchup, salad dressing, mayonnaise, peanut butter, cereal bars, and juices. High sugar consumption is associated with numerous health problems. Studies have linked diets high in refined sugar to diabetes, obesity, elevated triglycerides (a type of blood fat), tooth decay, poor immune function, and allergies. Plus, high-sugar foods are typically higher in the glycemic index, and we know what that can do to us. Excess sugar consumption has become such a serious health concern that the World Health Organization recently recommended reducing sugar intake to below 10 percent of total calories. For a person consuming 2,000 calories per day, this would represent 12 teaspoons of sugar per day.

Sugar Addiction

Sugar or sweet cravings are often driven by imbalances in blood sugar levels. The body gets used to, and begins to depend on, a regular supply of refined sugar. When blood sugar is low, which occurs an hour or so after a high-GI meal, we crave more sweets. Even though the body does not respond well to high blood sugar levels, it also naturally seeks balance. Overindulging in sweets can affect both physical and emotional well-being, causing headaches, fatigue, mood swings, irritability, anxiety, and impaired mental function.

Sweeter Alternatives

For better health, minimize your intake of refined sugar. If you crave something sweet, have a piece of fruit such as an apple or pear. Dried fruits provide concentrated sources of vitamins and minerals along with fiber, and many are low to moderate on the GI, such as apricots, dates, and prunes. Instead of using white sugar, try sweetening your foods with honey, maple syrup, malt syrups, or date sugar. These products provide some nutritional value and are not as hard on blood sugar levels as refined sugar. In baked goods, mashed bananas and pure apple sauce are great substitutes for sugar. Artificial sweeteners such as aspartame and saccharin should be avoided because they have been linked to various health problems. Here are some other products that you can consider to sweeten foods and beverages:

Stevia

Stevia is a plant native to South and Central America that is up to 300 times sweeter than sugar. It has garnered attention with the rise in demand for natural, low-sugar food alternatives. Stevia has a negligible effect on blood glucose and has even been shown in some research to enhance glucose tolerance, making it a good choice for diabetics and those following a low-GI diet. Aside from being a great sweetener, stevia also has shown promise in medical research for treating obesity and high blood pressure. In Canada and the US, stevia is sold as a dietary supplement and is available both in powder for baking and in liquid form. You will find stevia products in some grocery stores and health food stores. Stevia has undergone extensive animal testing for toxicity with no adverse effects found. As well, no birth defects have been seen in animal studies. However, since it has not been studied in pregnant women it would be advisable to avoid use during pregnancy.

Fructose

Fructose is a simple sugar found naturally in many foods such as

fruits, honey, and some root vegetables (beets, yams, sweet potatoes, and onions). Fructose is the sweetest naturally occurring sugar,
estimated to be twice as sweet as sucrose (table sugar). This means
less fructose can be used to achieve the same level of sweetness. Consequently, fewer calories are consumed from foods when fructose is
used instead of sucrose. Fructose is much lower in the GI compared
to table sugar and it does not cause a rapid rise and subsequent fall in
blood glucose levels. As with table sugar, fructose can be bought at the
grocery store and used as a sweetener in place of sucrose.

High-fructose corn syrup (HFCS) is a derivative of fructose in which
corn syrup undergoes enzymatic processing to convert it into a sweeter
product. HFCS is used widely in soft drinks, condiments, breads, cereals,
and many other foods. There are concerns with this sweetener as some
research has shown that it can trigger an appetite and addiction, and
it has been associated with obesity. It is probably best to minimize consumption of HFCS until more is known about its impact on health.

Xylitol

Xylitol is a naturally occurring sweetener found in the fibers of many
fruits and vegetables, including berries, corn husks, and oats. It is in
a group of sweeteners called sugar alcohols. Other sweeteners in this
group include sorbitol, mannitol, and maltitol. Xylitol is roughly as
sweet as sucrose, but with two-thirds the calories and a lesser impact
on blood sugar levels (lower GI). One teaspoon of xylitol contains
9.6 calories, compared to 1 teaspoon of sugar, which has 15 calories.
Xylitol also contains zero net effective carbohydrates, whereas sugar
contains 4 grams per teaspoon.

One benefit of xylitol (and other sugar alcohols) is that bacteria
in the mouth cannot use it as a source of energy. Therefore, they do
not contribute to dental caries (cavities). Xylitol has virtually no aftertaste and is now added to a variety of foods such as candy, chocolate,
table syrups, chewing gum, jams and jellies, and some cookies. Many

of these products are marketed to diabetics and those following low-GI diets because they have less of an impact on blood glucose levels. A drawback of using sugar alcohols is that they are only partially digested and metabolized, and therefore a high intake (greater than 10–20 grams per day) can cause flatulence, diarrhea, and upset stomach.

The Lowdown of Low-Carb Diets

Low-carb diets are based on the premise that without sufficient glucose for energy, the body will burn its fat stores for energy. As such, in the short term at least, low-carb diets help encourage weight loss. Several problems, though, are associated with cutting carbs from the diet.

Low-carb diets deprive the cells of their primary energy source (glucose). When this happens, the body uses glycogen stored in the liver and converts it into glucose. Once glycogen is depleted, the body converts fat and protein into glucose for a source of fuel. The use of protein, which comes from muscle, can result in muscle wasting (loss). When fat is used to provide energy, the liver takes fatty acids and produces compounds called ketone bodies. This is known as ketosis. Some consider ketosis to be a sign of dieting success. However, if the brain is utilizing ketones for energy (instead of proper glucose), then it is not working at its best and mental function may decrease (that is, it may result in sluggishness, depression, impaired judgment, and impaired memory). The brain is the most energy-intensive organ in the body, responsible for over half our energy requirements. The benefits of carbs on mental performance are well documented. Long-term low-carb dieting can impair brain and nervous system function.

Another major concern is that low-carb diets often result in deficiencies of vitamins, minerals, and essential fatty acids because these nutrients are obtained from eating vegetables, fruits, and whole grains, which are restricted on a low-carb diet.

Lastly, a low-carb diet can be very difficult to follow. And when you start eating carbs again, the weight comes back, and you may even gain more weight than you started with. This frustration may lead to yo-yo dieting or more drastic forms of dieting.

Due to the concerns about low-carb diets and the necessity of carbohydrates for brain function, the Institute of Medicine recommended that adults consume a minimum of 130 grams of carbohydrates daily. This would be the equivalent of eating a bowl of bran flakes with milk and berries in the morning, a sandwich on whole-grain bread at lunch, an apple for a snack, and then vegetables and brown rice for dinner. Most people exceed the recommended amount and consume 200–330 grams per day.

The Power of Protein

Protein is in animal products (meat and dairy), nuts, legumes, and, to a lesser extent, in grains and vegetables. Protein is a necessary component for building, maintaining, and repairing many bodily systems and processes. Protein is required for:

- Production of collagen and keratin, which are the structural components of bones, teeth, hair, and the outer layer of skin; collagen and keratin maintain the structure of blood vessels

- Production of hormones, such as insulin and thyroid hormone

- Production of enzymes that control chemical reactions in the body

- Production of antibodies, white blood cells, and other immune factors

- Transportation of oxygen, vitamins, and minerals to target cells throughout the body

- Provision of a secondary source of energy when there are not enough carbohydrates available, such as when you skip a meal or avoid carbs

Proteins are broken down during digestion into amino acids, some of which are called *essential* because they must be provided by the food we eat. Others that can be produced by the body are called *nonessential.*

Animal source protein contains all of the essential amino acids. Therefore, your best sources of lean protein are chicken, turkey, fish, and eggs. Choose free-range and organic whenever possible to reduce ingesting harmful hormones and chemicals. Red meat should be eaten less frequently (once or twice a week) because it is high in saturated fat.

Plant proteins do not contain all the essential amino acids and are considered *incomplete* proteins. It is possible, however, to combine various plant proteins to get all the essential amino acids. For example, eating oats, lentils, and sunflower seeds either together or separately throughout the day provides all the essential amino acids. You could also combine whole-wheat pasta with white kidney beans or tofu with brown rice to get all the necessary amino acids. It just requires careful meal planning.

There are certain advantages to eating plant over animal protein: Plant proteins provide fiber and phytochemicals (antioxidants), do not contain saturated fat, and may play a role in disease prevention. Soy protein, for example, has been shown to significantly lower cholesterol and triglyceride levels, and to protect against bone loss. A number of studies have found lower risk of chronic diseases in those who eat a plant-based diet.

Boost Your Metabolism, Lower the GI

When we eat protein, it raises our metabolic rate to a greater extent than eating just carbohydrates or fat alone. As a result you will burn more calories! Eating protein with carbohydrates in a meal can also help keep insulin and blood sugar levels under control because protein slows down the rate of digestion of carbohydrates. Thus it has the effect of lowering the overall glycemic impact of your meal.

Too Much of a Good Thing

As noted in the beginning of this chapter, the Institute of Medicine recommends that adults get 10–35 percent of calories from protein. Protein provides 4 calories per gram, so for a person consuming a 2,000-calorie-day diet, the target range would be 50–175 grams per day.

Protein deficiency is rare, except among vegetarians, the elderly, and those engaging in heavy exercise (exercise increases protein requirements). A more common concern, though, is consuming too much protein. Protein powders, bars, and supplements have become popular beyond the body-building circle. It is a common misconception that protein can't make you fat. Excess protein cannot be stored by the body; instead, it is broken down into amino acids. The liver removes nitrogen from the amino acids, so that they can be burned as fuel, and the nitrogen is incorporated into urea, which is excreted by the kidneys. Excess amino acids are converted into sugars and fatty acids and if not utilized for energy, they can be stored as fat, so excess protein can indeed make you fat. But the problems don't end here. Excess protein can also be hard on your kidneys and liver. The kidneys can normally cope with an extra workload, but if a person has kidney disease, this excess can be a problem. Excessive protein intake may also cause the body to lose calcium, which could lead to bone loss over time. It can also be harmful (toxic) to the liver and cause an overreactive immune system.

Fats: The Good and the Bad

"Fat" has become a negative word as it is associated with obesity, yet we do need a certain amount of fat in our diets and on our bodies. It is important, though, to make a distinction between the *good* fats and *bad* fats. Consuming the right amount of good fats and avoiding bad fats will greatly improve your overall health and weight-loss efforts.

Good Fats

The good fats are the unsaturated fats, namely, the monounsaturated fats (olive, canola, and peanut oil) and polyunsaturated fats. The poly-unsaturated fats provide us with essential fatty acids (EFAs), which are broken down into two groups, the omega-3 and omega-6 fatty acids.

Omega-3 fatty acids are found in fatty fish, such as salmon, mackerel, herring, cod, sardines, and tuna. These fats are also found to a lesser extent in flaxseed and hemp oil, and in nuts, green leafy vegetables, wheat germ, and black currant seeds.

Omega-6 fatty acids are found in vegetable oils, such as safflower, sunflower, corn, hemp, canola, and olive oil. It is also found in supplements of borage, black currant, and evening primrose oil.

The body cannot make EFAs, so they must be obtained through diet or supplementation. They are essential for many body processes and functions:

- Growing and developing brain, nervous system, adrenal glands, sex organs, the inner ear, and eyes
- Providing energy (fat is the most concentrated source of energy)
- Absorbing fat-soluble vitamins (carotenoids vitamins A, D, E, K)
- Maintaining cell membrane integrity
- Regulating cell processes such as gene activation and expression, enzyme function, and fat oxidation
- Producing hormones and chemical messengers

There is great controversy over what is the optimal dietary intake ratio of omega-6 to omega-3 fatty acids. It is estimated that we consume 10–20 times more omega-6s than omega-3s.

Rather than trying to calculate the perfect ratio or intake, aim to have more omega-3s (fish, flaxseed, hemp, and seed oils) from diet and/or supplements as these are the fats that are commonly deficient, yet offer a number of health benefits. Since the majority of our fish supply (particularly salmon) is contaminated with toxic chemicals, health authorities recommend limiting intake of farmed and even wild fish. Quality fish oil supplements are readily available and provide concentrated amounts of the beneficial omega-3 fatty acids (EPA and DHA) without the contaminants.

Diets rich in the omega-3 fatty acids offer heart protection by lowering blood cholesterol and triglyceride levels, reducing blood clotting, and reducing the risk of heart attack and sudden death. These fats also reduce inflammation and are helpful for arthritis and other inflammatory disorders. Omega-6 fatty acids help reduce inflammation, prevent clotting, dilate blood vessels, improve skin health, and are beneficial to those with diabetes and arthritis.

Fat Free Frenzy

There is great confusion surrounding fats. Many dieters think that in order to lose body fat you need to cut out dietary fat. This is simply not true. Good fats (essential fatty acids) can actually help support your weight loss efforts by reducing body fat storage and boosting metabolism (helping your body burn calories more efficiently). Cutting fat from the diet has serious consequences: depression, hair loss, and skin irritation. Taking fats out of the diet and substituting them with carbs can also make you fat! In fact, as a result of the low-fat craze in the 1980s, many food manufacturers reduced the fat content of their foods (creating low-fat sour cream, yogurt, and snacks, for example). However, in order to keep these foods palatable they substituted the fat with starch and sugar. So rather than becoming healthier, many of these foods became high GI and contained just as many calories as the original product. And rather than lose weight, we became fatter. So don't be fooled by low-fat marketing. In many cases the low-fat version is no better for you.

Bad Fats

Saturated fats and trans fats should be limited or completely avoided in the diet if possible. Below is an explanation of these fats and why they are harmful to our health.

Saturated Fats

Saturated fats are in animal products such as meat, poultry, milk, cheese, butter, and lard, as well as in tropical oils (such as palm, palm kernel, and coconut oil) and foods made from these oils. A diet high in saturated fat is linked to heart disease, high cholesterol, obesity, and cancers of the breast, colon, and prostate. However, there are some key differences among the saturated fats.

Butter, coconut oil, and palm kernel oil are classified as short-chain saturated fats. They are easily digested, provide a source of energy, and do not clog arteries. The bad saturates are those found in red meat and the trans fats, which are discussed below.

Most people get 38 percent or more of the day's calories from fat, while health authorities suggest no more than 20–35 percent, of which less than 10 percent is saturated fat. To cut your intake of saturated fat, trim fat and skin from meat, choose lean poultry over red meat, avoid deep-frying foods, and choose low-fat cheese and dairy (cottage cheese, feta, and hard cheeses have less saturated fat). Butter is fine in moderation (1–2 teaspoons per day).

Trans Fats

Trans fatty acids are naturally found in small amounts in animal products. However, the majority of trans fats in our diet come from commercial foods. Trans fats are created when oils undergo a chemical process called hydrogenation, which changes them from a liquid into a solid form. This is the process that turns vegetable oil into margarine. Trans fats are also found in cookies, crackers, french fries, baked goods, and other processed and snack foods.

When trans fats were first introduced into our food supply, they were thought to be a healthier alternative to saturated fats. Many years later this was found to be false. Trans fats elevate cholesterol levels, increasing the risk for heart disease and heart attack, and are also linked to cancer, particularly breast cancer. The Institute of Medicine has stated that there is no safe limit for trans fats in the diet, and that we should reduce consumption of these dangerous fats. Food companies have been making efforts in this area. You will now see many packaged foods labelled "trans fat free." Read food labels carefully and avoid consuming products that contain hydrogenated oils.

Cholesterol

Cholesterol is a waxy substance found in the fats (lipids) in our blood. It is manufactured in the liver and also obtained from consuming saturated and trans fats.

Approximately 75 percent of the body's cholesterol is produced in the liver, and the rest is obtained from diet. While having elevated blood cholesterol levels is a risk factor for heart disease, the news on cholesterol is not all bad—the body requires it to produce sex hormones, to maintain cell membranes, and for a healthy nervous system.

In addition to diet, cholesterol levels can be elevated by family history (genetics), lack of activity, stress, and liver disorders.

As with fats, there is good and bad when it comes to cholesterol. LDL (low-density lipoproteins) cholesterol is called *bad* because it can build up in the artery walls of the brain and heart, narrowing the passageways for blood flow, a process known as atherosclerosis, the precursor to heart disease and stroke.

HDL (high-density lipoproteins) cholesterol is called *good* cholesterol because it picks up the LDL deposited in the arteries and transports it to the liver to be broken down and eliminated.

To lower LDL and raise HDL levels, exercise regularly, minimize saturated fats, avoid trans fats, and don't smoke (smoking lowers HDL).

Triglycerides

Triglycerides (TG) are the form in which most fats exist. They are also present in the blood along with cholesterol.

A diet that is high in fat, sugar, refined carbohydrates, and alcohol can elevate TGs. Overeating also raises TG levels because excess calories are converted to fat in the liver and then into TGs to be transported in the blood. High levels of triglycerides are associated with heart disease and diabetes. It is possible for triglycerides to be high even when blood cholesterol is normal, so get your levels checked regularly. In most cases, TG levels can be effectively managed with diet and exercise.

———•◦•◦•———

As you can see, there are many factors to consider for good nutrition and effective weight loss. The glycemic index is one of those factors, but following a low-GI diet alone will not ensure successful weight loss. It is also important to choose quality proteins and fats that will improve the glycemic load or impact of your meals and support overall health.

Now that we understand the components of good nutrition, it is time to look at other aspects of a successful health program, namely, exercise, sleep, and stress management.

5
EXERCISE, SLEEP, AND DESTRESS FOR SUCCESS

$\mathcal{E}$ating a low-GI diet is crucial for glycemic control and will certainly help facilitate weight loss, but it works best when we take a broader view of our health. Other lifestyle factors that play an important role, include exercise, sleep, and stress management. Let's see how we can develop a multipronged strategy for success.

Exercise For a Leaner Body and Better Health

There are many reasons why exercise is particularly helpful for weight loss and glycemic control. Firstly, it's the most effective way to boost metabolism (the rate of calorie burning). Your basal (resting) metabolic rate is heightened for four to 24 hours after vigorous physical activity. Secondly, exercise builds and maintains strong, healthy muscles. Muscle burns more calories than any other part of the body. Consider this: 1 pound of muscle burns approximately 50 calories per day, compared to a pound of fat, which burns only 2–3 calories per day. Exercise can also help control appetite by slowing down the passage of food through the digestive tract, so that your stomach takes longer to empty and you feel full longer.

With respect to blood sugar control, physical activity helps your muscle cells use blood glucose for energy, and it makes those cells more sensitive to insulin (improving insulin resistance). Many studies have shown that regular exercise can help prevent type 2 diabetes. In some diabetics, it may even reduce the need for medication. In a report from the Ottawa Health Research Institute, researchers did a comprehensive review of clinical studies that looked at the effects of at least eight weeks of exercise on adults with type 2 diabetes. They determined that regular exercise did in fact reduce the risk of diabetic complications by lowering blood sugar levels.

The benefits of exercise extend to many other aspects of health. Consider these other impressive rewards:

- *Better sleep:* Studies have shown that exercise can improve sleep quality.

- *Enhanced longevity:* Regular physical activity lowers the risk of premature death from all causes.

- *Improved energy:* Believe it or not, regular exercise can actually make you feel more energized.

- *Improved mood:* Even light exercise can boost your emotional well-being. Aerobic exercise stimulates the release of certain mood-elevating compounds called endorphins, "feel good" chemicals. These natural painkillers induce relaxation and relieve depression.

- *Increased bone density:* Activities that put stress on the bones (walking, weight training) stimulate bone growth and protect against bone loss. In one study, sedentary 90-year-old nursing home residents performed mild exercises for 30 minutes, three times a week. On average, they experienced a 4.2 percent increase in their bone density.

- *Increased mental acuity:* Physical activity can invigorate and revitalize the mind and improve the flow of blood, oxygen, and nutrients to all the body's organs, including the brain.

- *Increased strength:* The National Institutes of Health found that men and women aged 86–96 tripled the muscular strength of their legs when they worked out with weights.

- *Pain relief:* Exercise triggers the release of pain-reducing endorphins. Strength training and stretching can help decrease arthritis pain and improve joint flexibility.

ఈ *Reduced risk of heart disease:* Exercise can also effectively lower blood pressure and cholesterol, and facilitate weight loss, reducing risk factors for heart disease. In a study conducted at Washington University School of Medicine in St. Louis, Missouri a group of individuals participated in a 12-month exercise program that increased their cardiovascular function by 25–30 percent.

Creating Your Exercise Program

If you have been sedentary all your life, the prospect of getting active may be intimidating. The most important advice for beginners is to take it slowly. Where do you start? Three words: Just start moving. That may sound like an oversimplification, but it's amazing how hard it is to take those first steps. You need to look at exercise in the same way you do any other essential daily routine such as brushing your teeth or showering. Getting into shape is a gradual, incremental process. If you do too much too soon, you may injure yourself or become too discouraged to continue. For example, start by taking a five-minute walk. The next day, walk six or seven minutes. Day by day, steadily increase the time and intensity of your activity. You will build your capacity for physical activity, making it easier to push yourself to the next level. Once you get started, you will be amazed at how great you feel and how much more energy you have. Aim to do a combination of cardiovascular (aerobic) and stretching activities. Here is a breakdown of each of these activities and some guidelines to consider:

Cardiovascular (Aerobic) Exercise

Cardiovascular activities involve large muscle groups and increase heart rate for more than a few minutes. Examples include brisk walking, swimming, biking, aerobics, dancing, and in-line skating. These exercises help burn calories, and also improve cardiovascular and respiratory (lung) function by conditioning the lungs to be able to use more oxygen while increasing your heart's efficiency.

Aim for 30 minutes to one hour five times per week. Pick activities you enjoy and do them in the morning or right after work, preferably on an empty stomach. Morning is best because you will have more energy and will continue to burn calories for several hours afterward.

To increase intensity, add resistance or power to the movements. For example, when a brisk walk becomes easy, add hand weights or walk up hills. Moving your arms above your heart will also increase your heart rate.

Check Your Heart Rate

Aerobic activity should increase your heart rate to 60–80 percent of your maximum rate for 30 minutes or longer. To find your maximum rate, subtract your age from 220. For example, if you are 50 years old:

$220 - 50 = 170$

60–80 percent of 170 = 102–136

Divide by 6 to get the 10-second heartbeat count, which is 17–23.

For optimum aerobic benefits, keep your heart rate within this range for 30 minutes.

Resistance Training

Activities that challenge your muscles against resistance strengthen bones and increase strength, endurance, and muscle mass. This can be achieved with weight lifting, exercise machines, bands/tubes, using your own body weight, or lifting heavy objects. These activities are particularly important for older adults because they help prevent and slow the muscle and bone loss that occurs with aging.

Try to spend 20–30 minutes three to four times a week doing resistance activities. Choose two body parts per workout. For example, do chest and triceps on Monday, back and biceps on Wednesday, and legs and shoulders on Friday. Pick two exercises per body part and do two or three sets of 8–12 repetitions of that exercise. Vary your activities and routine to continually challenge your muscles.

Stretching

Stretching after a workout is a great way to improve flexibility and joint health and prevent next-day soreness. Spend about five to 10 minutes stretching all your muscles. This is also a great way to promote relaxation. Stretch slowly and gently, breathe deeply, and hold each position for at least 10 seconds.

How Much Exercise Do I Need?

Guidelines from the National Academy of Sciences and the Institute of Medicine (used in Canada and the United States) recommend that, regardless of weight, adults and children should spend a total of at least one hour each day in moderately intense physical activity. This recommendation takes into consideration the increased caloric intake of our population, our lack of activity, and our rising prevalence of obesity.

Building Activity into Your Day

Our modern way of life with automated, drive-through, express convenience, offers few opportunities for regular exercise. While you can certainly lose weight by reducing your calorie intake, regular exercise can greatly enhance your weight-loss program. Consider this: Adding a 30-minute brisk walk four days a week can double your rate of weight loss. Boost that to five days a week and the rewards are greater. Those who work out five times a week have been found to lose three times as much fat as those who exercise only two or three times weekly.

If you don't have an hour that you can dedicate to exercise, work on incorporating more activity into your daily routine. Every little bit helps. Studies have actually shown that the benefits of exercise are cumulative (that is, performing 10 minutes of exercise several times a day is as effective as performing all the exercise at once). Here are some suggestions:

- Do housework or gardening with vim and vigor.
- Take the stairs instead of the elevator.
- Use your break at work to go for a brisk walk.
- Ride your bike to the store.
- Park your car farther away and walk to your destination.
- Wash your car instead of using the drive-through.

Take Pride in Your Progress

Even modest weight loss can yield impressive health benefits. A weight loss of even 5–10 percent has been shown to help prevent diabetes, reduce blood pressure and cholesterol, and improve quality of life.

The Significance of Sleep

Sleep is one of our bodies' most basic needs, yet with today's busy lifestyles it often gets sacrificed. Sleep deprivation has become all too common. In fact, nearly half of all North American adults report having difficulty sleeping. While we think of sleep as a relaxing and passive state, there is actually quite a lot going on in our bodies during sleep. This is the time when our bodies repair, regenerate, and produce various hormones and chemicals.

The exact amount of sleep needed varies among individuals, but is thought to be between seven and nine hours. Getting less than six hours is associated with health problems such as memory loss, poor concentration, depression, headache, irritability, increased response to stress, high blood pressure, depressed immune function, and low libido.

Recently, sleep deprivation has been linked to weight gain and obesity. Several studies have shown that getting less than six hours per night can lead to hormonal changes that reduce metabolism and increase appetite, factors that lead to weight gain. Specifically, lack of sleep increases the level of a hormone called ghrelin. It is involved in appetite regulation and increased levels can increase appetite. Also, human growth hormone (HGH) is reduced when we don't get enough sleep. HGH is involved in regulating metabolism, so when levels of this hormone are lowered, this can reduce metabolism. In one study, participants who slept five hours per night were 73 percent more likely to become obese than those getting seven to nine nightly hours of sleep. So for better appetite and weight control, don't skimp on sleep.

Strategies for Better Sleep

To improve sleep quality, develop a good bedtime routine. Try to go to bed at approximately the same time each night. Make your bedroom quiet, comfortable, and dark and use it only for sleep (don't work in bed). Do relaxing activities in the evening—read a book, have a warm bath, enjoy a cup of chamomile tea, or meditate. Avoid exercising before bed as this can be stimulating and affect your ability to fall asleep. Caffeinated beverages (soft drinks, coffee, and tea) should be avoided four hours before bedtime. While alcohol may make you drowsy, it reduces your ability to stay asleep and affects sleep quality.

If you have difficulty getting a good night's rest, there are a variety of natural sleep aids that can be helpful, including:

- ⁊ Lactium®, a supplement derived from milk protein that promotes calming and relaxation and helps improve sleep. The usual dosage is 167 milligrams per day, taken at bedtime.

- ⁊ Melatonin, a hormone naturally secreted by the brain in response to darkness; it regulates sleep/wake cycles. This supplement is most helpful for people who work shifts or travel to different time zones. The typical dosage is 3–6 milligrams before bed.

ⁱ Suntheanine®, an extract of theanine (amino acid present in green tea). It helps improve sleep quality and reduce stress. The dosage is 50–100 milligrams 30 minutes before bed.

ⁱ Valerian, a herb that is widely used for insomnia. It improves many aspects of sleep and is nonaddictive. Some formulas combine valerian with hops, passionflower, and other herbs that promote relaxation. The usual dosage is 600 milligrams half an hour to one hour before bed, or 2 millilitres of a tincture.

Did You Know?

Snacking before bedtime, especially on refined carbohydrates, can have a negative impact on sleep. High-GI foods, such as soda crackers and rice cakes, will raise insulin levels. High insulin levels can reduce the action of melatonin, the sleep-inducing hormone.

Surviving Stress

Stress is a primary cause of many health problems today. According to recent reports, 43 percent of all adults suffer the adverse health effects of stress, and stress-related ailments account for 75–90 percent of all visits to physicians. Stress is not an external force, but rather how we react to external pressures. During stress, the body releases stress hormones—adrenaline, noradrenaline, and cortisol—to prepare the body to fight, so this is known as the fight or flight response. Heart rate, blood pressure, and lung function increase to enhance the function of the heart and lungs. Numerous studies have linked stress to heart disease, cancer, diabetes, high cholesterol and blood pressure, anxiety, depression, memory loss, insomnia, muscle tension, obesity, fatigue, low libido, erectile dysfunction, and menstrual cycle disturbances.

In recent years, many studies have looked at the connection between stress and obesity. Researchers have found that chronic stress causes weight gain due to a number of factors. Chronic stress increases the production of the hormone cortisol, which promotes fat storage, primarily around the belly. Stress also reduces insulin sensitivity and causes hormonal changes that trigger cravings for carbohydrates and sweets. Lastly, stress can lead to muscle wasting, which reduces metabolism.

For weight-loss success, work on reducing your stress. Start by identifying your stressors and then look at ways to change your reaction to those situations. It may be a matter of analyzing and rethinking your natural reaction, avoiding certain situations, or utilizing some of the following stress-reducing strategies:

- *Avoid negativity:* Negative people, places, and events can create stress.

- *Body therapies:* Try massage, acupuncture, and acupressure to promote relaxation of the body and mind.

- *Boundaries:* Learn to say "no." Taking on too much leads to feeling overwhelmed and pressed for time.

- *Meditation:* Sit down in a quiet area and close your eyes. Relax all your muscles, starting with your feet and working up. Clear your mind and focus your attention on your breathing or a calming sight or sound. Breathe in slowly and deeply, and then exhale. Do this for 10 to 20 minutes once or twice daily.

- *Supplements:* There are a variety of natural products that can help support the body during stress and promote relaxation, including Suntheanine (amino acid from green tea), Lactium (milk protein supplement), B-vitamins, and magnesium.

- *Talk about it:* Share your feelings and concerns, and get support from friends, family, or a therapist.

- *Visualization:* Close your eyes, take a few deep breaths, and visualize a picture or event that made you feel calm and centered. Focus on the details, sounds, images, and smells.

As you can see, successful weight loss and blood sugar control requires a comprehensive strategy that includes some lifestyle changes. These changes may require a bit of work initially, but the rewards will be worth it because you will experience better physical and emotional health.

Now let's take a look at the role of nutritional supplements and how they can give you an edge and support your overall program.

6
NUTRITIONAL SUPPLEMENTS

*A*s a pharmacist, I am always skeptical about weight-loss products, especially those that make outrageous claims. Of the numerous weight-loss products on the market promising to help you shed weight, few have been clinically tested for safety, let alone tested to see whether or not they work.

Weight loss is not easy and there is no magic bullet. If there were, then we would not have such a problem with obesity. However, there are a handful of supplements that have been shown in clinical studies to offer various benefits. Finding the right supplement can help the following:

- Control sugar cravings
- Curb your appetite
- Enhance your metabolism
- Improve blood sugar control
- Prevent the storage of fat
- Promote lean muscle mass
- Reduce starch digestion

All of the supplements listed in this chapter have undergone clinical testing. However, it is always good to consult with your doctor or pharmacist before taking any new medication or supplement to make sure that it is right for you. Now, let's take a look at my top recommended supplements.

Phase 2®

Phase 2 is a standardized extract taken from the white kidney bean. It promotes weight loss and improves glycemic control by reducing starch digestion. Phase 2 works in the intestine by temporarily inhibiting the activity of alpha amylase, the enzyme that breaks down starch into smaller glucose (sugar) molecules. As a result, fewer starch calories are absorbed from a meal and it reduces the rise in blood sugar that occurs after we've eaten starchy foods. As you now know, foods high in starch include many of our favorites that can be moderate or high GI, such as bread, pasta, potatoes, rice, and baked goods. Phase 2 is good news for those of us who are serious about using the GI to promote weight loss and health. It is still important though to choose healthy carbohydrates with a high nutrient value.

Research on Phase 2

In clinical studies, Phase 2 has been shown to lower blood sugar levels after a meal, reduce the amount of starch absorbed, and promote loss of body fat.

In two of the initial studies on Phase 2, participants were given a standardized meal containing 60 grams of starch (four slices of white bread) and either a placebo or 1,500 milligrams of Phase 2 in a margarine spread. After the meal, participants who were given Phase 2 had an average 66 percent reduction in after-meal blood sugar levels compared to the placebo group. Participants given Phase 2 reported no adverse side effects in either study.

An independent study conducted in Italy was the first to show that supplementing with Phase 2 could lead to substantial weight loss. This double-blind, placebo-controlled study involved 60 overweight individuals aged 25–45. Participants ate starchy foods during one of their principal meals, and took their test product (Phase 2 or a placebo) at that time. Researchers measured body weight; body fat percentage; and hip, waist, and thigh circumference. By the end of the 30-day study period, participants who took the Phase 2 lost an average of 6.5 pounds and 10.5 percent fat mass and had significant reductions in all body measurements compared to those in the placebo group, who lost little or no weight

A study conducted at Northridge Hospital Medical Center (University of California, Los Angeles), and published in *Alternative Medicine Review*, found that participants given Phase 2 lost an average of 4 pounds in eight weeks, had an average 26-point reduction in triglycerides, and had greater energy. Those participants given a placebo lost only 1.6 pounds.

Other weight-loss studies with Phase 2 have been conducted in Mexico, Japan, and the United States, yielding impressive and significant results. Most recently this supplement was found to lower the glycemic index of starchy foods. The clinical evidence on Phase 2 is so significant that it is allowed to be sold with a claim for weight control.

Phase 2 is particularly helpful for those struggling with obesity and diabetes as well as metabolic syndrome, or those looking to improve glycemic control and insulin resistance. It allows people to eat starchy foods while minimizing the amount of starch (sugar) absorbed. Phase 2 is safe and well tolerated and is not known to interact with any drugs or supplements. The recommended dosage of Phase 2 is 1,000–1,500 milligrams before starchy meals. Phase 2 is available in a variety of forms, including tablets, capsules, and soft chews. It is also being incorporated into baked goods under the name Starchlite™.

PGX™

PGX (PolyGlycopleX) is a blend of highly purified, naturally occurring, soluble fibers. In clinical studies, it has been shown to regulate after-meal blood glucose levels, lower blood cholesterol, reduce appetite and food cravings, improve fat burning and increase insulin sensitivity for reduced fat storage.

When added to liquid, PGX absorbs 600 times its weight in water. In fact, PGX is approximately seven times as viscous as psyllium. If it is taken with adequate liquid, it will expand in the stomach and intestine and keep appetite under control for several hours by providing a sense of fullness.

Research on PGX

The Canadian Centre for Functional Medicine in British Columbia conducted a weight-loss evaluation study from December 2003 through February 2004. It found that participants following the center's prescribed weight-loss program, which included PGX, lost up to 2 pounds per week, primarily body fat, and maintained lean muscle mass. Besides reversing insulin resistance, PGX helps normalize important appetite hormones and cholesterol levels. Research on PGX was presented at the American Diabetes Association's annual meeting in June 2004.

The recommended dosage is two to four capsules before meals with at least 8–16 ounces of water. PGX is also available in powder form.

Cinnamon

This popular spice has gained recent attention due to its bioactive compounds that offer a range of health benefits. The active ingredient in cinnamon is a water-soluble polyphenol compound called MHCP. In test tube experiments, MHCP mimics insulin, activates its receptor, and works synergistically with insulin in cells.

Research on Cinnamon

A 2003 study from the US Department of Agriculture's Human Nutrition Center found that a 1/2 teaspoon of cinnamon a day significantly reduced blood sugar levels in diabetics. Volunteers with type 2 diabetes were given 1, 3, or 6 grams of cinnamon powder a day after meals. All participants achieved blood sugar levels that were on average 20 percent lower than those in a control group. Some even achieved normal blood sugar levels.

Cinnulin PF® is a blend containing standardized amounts of the active compound found in cinnamon. In addition to supporting healthy glucose metabolism, the compound in Cinnulin PF has been shown to help optimize healthy cholesterol levels and bolster healthy blood pressure.

Sprinkle cinnamon on favorite foods such as yogurt, cereal, or toast. Or consider taking a cinnamon supplement, available from health food stores and pharmacies.

Conjugated Linoleic Acid (CLA)

CLA is a derivative of linoleic acid, which is a fatty acid found naturally in certain foods, such as meat and dairy products. Supplements of CLA are made from sunflower oil. Studies have shown that CLA can improve fat metabolism and maintain or improve lean muscle mass. Specifically, it works by increasing lipolysis (fat breakdown) and enhancing fatty acid oxidation (promotes burning of fat).

Research on CLA

The most widely studied CLA product on the market is Tonalin® CLA. Several clinical studies have found that this supplement can promote fat loss and prevent fat storage. A one-year, double-blind study compared Tonalin CLA and a placebo in 157 overweight adults. Researchers measured the participants' body fat mass and lean body mass. No changes were made to exercise or diet. At the end of the study it was found that a daily intake of 3.4 grams of Tonalin CLA produced an average 9 percent reduction in body fat mass and a small increase in lean body mass.

Subsequent to this study, 134 of the 157 participants volunteered to continue on in order to determine the long-term safety of the product and whether they could maintain their fat loss. They continued to take a dosage of 3.4 grams of Tonalin CLA per day for an additional 12 months. No serious adverse effects were reported and it was found that the participants were able to maintain their initial fat loss.

Most recently, a study was done during a holiday period to determine if Tonalin could prevent typical holiday weight gain. Forty overweight adults participated in this study. They were given either a placebo or 3.2 grams of Tonalin CLA daily. The researchers measured body composition before, during, and after the study. Those given the Tonalin CLA lost body fat during the study period, whereas those who were given a placebo gained weight. This study was published in the *International Journal of Obesity*, August 2006.

The recommended dosage of Tonalin is 4 grams daily, which provides 3.4 grams of actual CLA. While butter, whole milk, cheese, and beef contain some CLA, it would be difficult to get the recommended amount from these foods, and consuming large amounts of them is not recommended because of their saturated fat content. CLA is well tolerated and there are no known drug interactions.

Advantra Z®

Advantra Z is a patented extract of *citrus aurantium* (bitter orange), which has been studied for its weight-loss effects. Advantra Z contains compounds that work together to increase thermogenesis, or the rate of calorie burning.

Citrus aurantium is chemically similar to ephedra (a once popular weight-loss aid that has been removed from the market due to serious adverse effects), but has different effects in the body. *Citrus aurantium* selectively stimulates beta-3 cell receptors, which are located primarily in the fatty tissue and the liver. Stimulation of these receptors activates lipolysis (fat breakdown) and thermogenesis (fat burning). It may also give your workouts more clout. By releasing free fatty acids during aerobic exercise, this supplement may help provide more energy, thereby facilitating improved physical performance.

Research on Advantra Z

Research conducted at McGill University's Nutrition and Food Science

Centre in Montreal found that Advantra Z increased the thermogenic effect of food (TEF), meaning that the subjects burned more calories and stored less fat. The supplement was also well tolerated, with no adverse effect on heart rate or blood pressure. Earlier studies also found that citrus aurantium had comparable thermogenic effects to ephedra, but without the side effects commonly associated with ephedra use.

There have been some concerns raised about citrus aurantium, as a few reports suggested that it could increase blood pressure. However, an evaluation of these reports revealed that most of the cases involved either ephedra alone or in combination with citrus aurantium and no direct causal relationship could be determined.

In a recent study the cardiovascular effects of Advantra Z were tested on a group of 23 overweight adults. Subjects were given a dose of 52 milligrams of Advantra Z along with 704 milligrams of caffeine and their heart rate and blood pressure were measured. No adverse effects on heart rate or blood pressure were noted; however, fat oxidation did increase in certain individuals.

Green Tea

Green tea has achieved worldwide recognition for its numerous health benefits. It has been shown to lower cholesterol and blood pressure, protect against certain cancers, block bacteria and viruses, improve digestion, and reduce the risk of ulcers and strokes. Green tea also helps to support weight loss. It provides a source of caffeine (about 20–50 milligrams per cup), a known thermogenic agent. Green tea is also rich in catechins, a type of antioxidant. In preliminary research, the combination of these ingredients has been found to help promote weight loss by burning more fat calories.

Research on Green Tea

A handful of studies have evaluated the weight-loss potential of green tea. In 2002, researchers at the National Institute of Health and Medical

Research in Marseille, France, reported the results of a study of a green tea extract in 70 moderately obese adults (90 percent women) ranging in age from 20–69. The patients took a standardized green tea extract providing 375 milligrams of green tea catechins per day for three months. Waist circumference decreased by an average of 4.5 percent and body weight was reduced by an average of 4.6 percent.

Researchers at the University of Geneva studied the effects of green tea on energy expenditures (calorie burning) in a small group of 10 healthy young men. For six weeks, the men took two capsules at each meal consisting of one of the following: green tea extract plus 50 milligrams of caffeine, 50 milligrams of caffeine alone, or a placebo. The participants followed a routine weight-maintenance diet. Three times during the study, they spent 24 hours in a special room where their respiration and energy expenditures were measured. Energy expenditures were 4 percent higher for men taking green tea extract compared to those taking caffeine or placebo. The researchers also found that men taking the green tea extract used more fat calories for energy than those taking a placebo. There was no difference between the caffeine users and the placebo users in terms of either overall calorie burning or fat calorie burning. The researchers concluded that the benefits seen in the green tea group cannot be explained by caffeine intake alone. They suggested that the caffeine interacted with the flavonoids in green tea to alter the body's use of norepinephrine, a chemical transmitter in the nervous system, and to increase the rate of calorie burning. Green tea did not affect the heart rate in the study participants.

For those who are looking at the general health benefits of green tea, studies have found benefits with ranges between 3 and 10 cups or more daily. Green tea can also be taken in capsule or tablet form. The usual recommended dosage is one tablet or capsule, three to four times daily, of a product that provides 90 milligrams of EGCG (the catechin in green tea) and 50 milligrams of caffeine per dosage.

Although green tea is well tolerated, it should be used cautiously by those sensitive to caffeine, such as those with high blood pressure, kidney disease, insomnia, or increased intraocular (eye) pressure.

Green tea may offer some additional benefits for weight management. Theanine, which is an amino acid present in green tea, has become a popular stress-reducing supplement. Studies conducted on the Suntheanine brand of theanine have found that it can promote calming and relaxation without causing sedation or memory loss, which can occur with prescription sedatives. Since stress raises cortisol, and elevated cortisol can lead to weight gain, this supplement may offer some benefits. Suntheanine may also be effective in curbing stress-related eating, such as cravings and binge eating, by modulating hormones. The recommended dosage is 50–200 milligrams twice or three times daily.

Chromium

Chromium is an essential trace mineral found in a wide variety of foods. It plays a significant role in the body by helping to regulate blood glucose. Chromium works along with insulin to move glucose into the cells to be used for energy.

A deficiency in chromium is very common in North America. According to some reports, 90 percent of individuals do not get enough through diet. The recommended dietary range is 50–200 micrograms daily. Inadequate chromium intake can cause impaired glucose tolerance and elevated blood glucose levels. It is thought that those with diabetes may have a deficiency of chromium.

Research on Chromium

In a double-blind, placebo-controlled study, 180 people with type 2 diabetes were given either 200 micrograms or 1,000 milligrams of chromium picolinate or a placebo daily. The researchers measured their HbA1c values (a measure of long-term blood sugar control) after two and four months. Participants who received 1,000 micrograms of chromium experienced a significant improvement after two months and both chromium groups had improvements after four months. Fasting glucose (a measure of short-term blood sugar control) was also lower in the group taking the higher dose of chromium.

Another double-blind study compared the effects of two different forms of chromium (brewer's yeast and chromium chloride) in 78 individuals with type 2 diabetes. After 32 weeks, all the participants who completed the study had significant improvement in blood sugar control, thus showing that both forms were effective in lowering blood sugar. Several other clinical trials have found chromium beneficial for people with type 2 diabetes. Chromium is also promoted for weight loss and fat burning, but the results in studies have been mixed.

Chromium is safe when taken at a dosage of up to 400 micrograms daily, and side effects are rare. At higher dosages, such as those taken for blood sugar control, it is recommended that you seek advice from your health care provider.

As you can see from the products discussed above, scientific research is critical. Testimonials and clever advertising do not mean that a product will work. Common sense must prevail. If a product sounds too good to be true, it usually is. Before taking any nutritional supplement, consult with your health care provider to see if there are any potential adverse reactions with medications that you may be taking. Find out about side effects and how to use the product properly, and remember—more is not always better. Some products can cause side effects, particularly if higher dosages are taken.

Nutritional Bars

Nutritional bars have become very popular among those with busy lifestyles as a convenient way to have small, nutritious meals throughout the day. They come in all sizes and flavors and with a wide range of purported benefits. It's important to keep in mind that not all bars are created equal. So how do you choose a good bar? Here are some factors to consider:

1. *Nutritional composition:* Look for a bar that provides wholesome ingredients (avoid products that contain artificial flavors and chemicals). Read the nutritional panel and look for a bar that provides 10–15 grams of protein (25–35 grams for body builders), 20–30 grams of carbohydrate (with at least 3 grams of fiber per serving), and 5–10 grams of fat, of which there are minimal saturated fats (less than 5 grams). Avoid products that contain trans fats (hydrogenated oils). Look for bars that provide a range of vitamins and minerals.

2. *Calories:* For a snack, choose a bar that provides 100–150 calories; for a meal replacement, look for a bar that provides 200–300 calories.

3. *Taste:* This is definitely an important consideration. Many bars have a chalky or unpleasant aftertaste. Taste is a matter of personal preference, so you may have to experiment with different brands until you find something you like.

4. *GI rating:* Most bars are moderate to high in the GI, and many have not even been tested. Be aware that many bars that are promoted as low carb are not necessarily low GI. Unless they have been tested for the GI, this is not something that can be assumed. Low-carb bars often contain sugar alcohols, such as malitol and xylitol instead of other sugar or other natural sweeteners. The problem is that in large amounts, sugar alcohols can cause diarrhea and gas.

With these points in mind, here are my top two recommended bars:

SoLo Gi™

SoLo Gi bars contain a unique combination of slow-release carbohydrates, protein, healthy fats, and fiber. This is the only bar that I am aware of that is rated as low GI. The bars are clinically validated to slowly release glucose into the blood over an extended period of time, preventing a spike and crash in blood sugar levels. This offers significant benefits—especially for people with diabetes, pre-diabetes, or metabolic syndrome—such as improved blood glucose levels, sustained energy, suppression of appetite, and the absence of food cravings. SoLo Gi bars have been included in various clinical trials, including two ongoing diabetes-related studies funded by the National Institutes of Health. These bars come in five different flavors and two sizes: snack bars (100 calories) and nutritional bars (200 calories). They do not contain any sugar alcohols, artificial sweeteners, trans fats, hydrogenated oils, or high-fructose corn syrup. Best of all, they taste great.

LARABAR®

These bars contain only dried fruits, nuts, and natural spices blended together. All of the vitamins, minerals, fiber, protein, good carbohydrates, and healthy fats are derived exclusively from the whole, raw ingredients. While they have not been tested yet for their GI, they would likely fare well as most dried fruits are low to moderate, and nuts provide protein and healthy fats, which help lower the glycemic impact. Larabar comes in 12 flavors, all gluten-free, dairy-free, and vegan. These bars also taste great.

There are many other many other quality bars on the market. It is important to read labels carefully when choosing a bar to see the composition and ingredients.

———•◦•◦•———

Keep in mind that a healthful, low-GI diet, along with regular exercise, adequate sleep, and stress management, is essential for healthy, long-term weight loss and improved blood sugar control. Use nutritional supplements and bars wisely to support, not replace, these lifestyle approaches. In the final chapter, I outline my recommendations for taking everything you've learned and putting it into action.

7
PUTTING IT ALL TOGETHER

$\mathcal{G}$ive yourself a pat on the back. You now know why proper blood sugar control and a low-glycemic diet is important for weight loss and overall health. Now you are ready to put it all together in your day-to-day life. This won't be as hard as you may think. I have put together a list of my top 10 dietary strategies to help you achieve success. You will also find a handy GI Food Chart, advice on shopping and stocking your pantry, tips on lowering the GI of your meals, and a 14-Day menu plan, along with some practical suggestions on eating out and surviving the holidays.

Top 10 Dietary Strategies

1. Reach for Fruits and Vegetables First

Fresh, natural, unprocessed fruits and vegetables should form the basis of your diet. Most are low GI, especially dark green vegetables, apples, pears, cherries, and berries. This tip may seem obvious, but it's the hardest one to implement, especially when you are tired, cold, hungry, or feeling blue, and tempted to grab a high-GI comfort food. Keep a good supply of fresh produce in your refrigerator so that these foods are easily accessible. Try yam, sweet potato, or taro as a low-GI substitute for potatoes. Experiment with new vegetables and try new recipes.

Don't dismiss certain fruits such as watermelon or mangos because they have a higher GI. All fruits provide a good source of vitamins, minerals, and fiber. Plus, remember that fruits and vegetables tend to have a low to moderate glycemic load because the amount of carbohydrates per serving is a factor. For example, a mango has a GI of 60 (moderate), but provides 15 grams of carbohydrate per serving, so the glycemic load is $(60 \times 15) \div 100 = 9$ (a low value). Just eat in moderation and watch your portion sizes—eating one mango won't have a dramatic effect on your blood sugar, but eating two or three most definitely will.

2. Choose Quality, Low-GI Grains

Remember that this is not a low-carb diet. The glycemic index allows you to choose a wide variety of carbohydrates at every meal. Choose whole grains over refined and processed products. By choosing low-GI carbs, you will achieve better blood sugar control and have less hunger, fewer cravings, and more energy.

Keep your pantry stocked with low-GI carbs, including different types of beans (chickpeas, lentils), sweet potatoes, old-fashioned oatmeal, muesli, and rolled oat cereals, whole-wheat or spinach pasta, basmati or whole-grain brown rice, plenty of fruits and vegetables, sourdough, pita, or whole-grain sprouted breads and whole-grain English muffins. These foods are also high in fiber so they can help fill you up.

Refined grains, such as white bread or bagels, processed cereals, and rice cakes, have had most of their nutrients and fiber stripped away during the refinement process. These foods are often high in sugar and calories, but low in nutritional value. If you enjoy these foods, have smaller portion sizes and eat them only occasionally. Pairing a high-GI food with a low-GI food can also help to lower the overall impact of the high-GI food, so mix the good with the bad. For example, have beans with your rice.

3. Include Protein and Healthy Fats in Every Meal

Proteins and fats are essential to a healthy, balanced diet, and also help to lower the glycemic impact of any given meal.

Protein is also vital for building and maintaining lean muscle mass. Without adequate protein, dieting and exercise can cause the body to burn muscle for fuel and this can result in a lowering of your basal metabolic rate, the rate at which you burn calories. Focus on eating lean protein, such as poultry, fish, eggs, nuts, seeds, and tofu. Red meat is okay in moderation, but be sure to trim the fat. If following a vegetarian diet, be sure to incorporate a variety of plant-based proteins to ensure that all essential amino acids are consumed. If you can't get enough protein in your diet, consider a protein supplement that provides at least 20 grams per serving, is low in carbohydrate, and free of artificial ingredients.

As discussed in Chapter 4, fats (essential fatty acids) are required for health. Good fats include fish, nuts, and seeds, and milled flax and hemp seed. Avoid saturated and trans fats, which are found in processed and fast foods, and research has linked them to heart disease and cancer. Plus, these fats fill you up more slowly because they take longer to metabolize and digest. Avoid the fat-free frenzy because many of the fat-free products (such as sour cream and yogurt) use sugar or starch in place of fat and end up providing just as many or more calories as the original product.

Butter vs. Margarine

Butter contains saturated fats, but they are short-chain saturates, which are easily digested and provide a source of usable energy. Butter also contains nutrients: lecithin, vitamins A and E, and selenium. Most margarine spreads contain hydrogenated oils (trans fats), which are artificially processed fats that are linked to heart disease and cancer. The exception is nonhydrogenated margarines, such as Becel™, which contain beneficial plant sterols that can help lower cholesterol. So the bottom line is: Choose butter or a nonhydrogenated margarine.

4. Enjoy a Variety of Wholesome Foods

To get a broad range of nutrients in your diet, enjoy a variety of foods, rather than sticking to your favorites. We have a tendency to eat the same foods over and over. By doing this, we miss out on some of the nutrients provided by eating different foods. This is particularly important with vegetables and fruits as their nutrient profiles vary greatly, even among low- to moderate-GI fruits and vegetables. To obtain the many antioxidants, vitamins, minerals, and phytonutrients available, eat a variety of plant foods every day. Experiment with new foods and recipes, and try foods that you previously disliked. Remember, our tastebuds change over time. You may have disliked spinach as a child, but give it another try.

5. Avoid Portion Distortion

Overeating can lead to obesity, high triglycerides, insulin resistance, free radical damage, and shortened life expectancy. To prevent overeating, control your portion sizes and eat slowly. A serving equals one piece of fruit, 1 cup of raw or 1/2 cup of cooked vegetables, one slice of bread, 1/2 cup of cooked rice or pasta, or 2–3 ounces of meat. Chew your food thoroughly and drink water to allow for proper digestion. Eating slowly allows your stomach to send a message to your brain that you are full. It should take you 20–30 minutes to eat a meal.

Caloric requirements are dependent upon your age, gender, height, weight, and activity level. The next chart shows average values for those 30 years and older.

6. Eat Small, Frequent Meals

Every day, try to eat three small meals and two snacks, with two to three hours between them. This will improve metabolism (calorie burning) and blood sugar balance, which improves energy and mood.

Breakfast is essential to fuel your body. If you aren't very hungry in the morning, then have a light meal such as yogurt and berries or a protein shake. Try not to eat too late in the evening (after 8 p.m.) as this could impact sleep. Don't skip meals, even if you are trying to lose weight, since this causes fatigue, poor concentration, and sluggish metabolism, and triggers food cravings. When you are hungry between meals, snack on healthy, low-GI foods, such as fruit, yogurt, raw vegetables, nuts, and seeds.

Height/Weight	Gender	Calories (Sedentary)	Calories (Active)
5'1" 98–132 pounds	Women	1,688–1,834	2,104–2,290
	Men	1,919–2,167	2,104–2,290
5'5" 111–150 pounds	Women	1,816–1,982	2,267–2,477
	Men	2,068–2,349	2,490–2,842
5'9" 125–169 pounds	Women	1,948–2,134	2,434–2,670
	Men	2,222–2,538	2,683–3,078
6'1" 139–188 pounds	Women	2,083–2,290	2,605–2,869
	Men	2,382–2,736	2,883–3,325

NOTE: Please consult you primary health care provider if you are pregnant, lactating, or engaged in vigorous physical activity.

Source: The Institute of Medicine of the National Academics (2006).

7. Go Easy on Salt

Salt (sodium) is necessary for health as it helps maintain fluid balance and aids muscle and nerve function. However, most people get more than twice the recommended amount of sodium. Foods high in sodium include processed and prepared foods, such as deli meats, condiments (ketchup), salad dressings and sauces (soy), and snack foods (chips, pretzels). Salty foods also tend to be bad choices because they are often processed and low in nutrient value.

A high-sodium diet causes fluid retention and can contribute to high blood pressure, especially in older individuals, African Americans, and those with diabetes and kidney disease, so cut back on these foods and season with herbs or flavored oils rather than the salt shaker. To add more zing to your meals, add fresh lemon juice or apple cider vinegar, which can lower the glycemic value of a meal by up to 30 percent.

8. Limit Caffeine and Alcohol

If you drink caffeinated beverages or alcohol, do so in moderation. Limit your intake to no more than 2 cups of caffeine daily. A high intake of caffeine can promote calcium loss from bones, increase blood pressure, affect fertility in women, and cause sleep disturbances (insomnia), anxiety, and tremors. Black tea and green tea contain some caffeine, but it's affects are blunted by an amino acid (theanine), which has a calming effect. Be on the lookout for hidden caffeine. Cola contains about 35 milligrams of caffeine per can. Chocolate contains 6–20 milligrams per ounce.

Alcohol floods the body with empty calories. Depending on the beverage, it provides 20–124 calories per ounce. Moderate alcohol consumption—no more than two glasses per day of red wine and dark beers—can reduce the risk of heart disease, likely due to its antioxidant content.

9. Drink More Water

One of the most important dietary tips I can give you is actually a simple one—drink plenty of pure water daily. Drinking water is critical for weight loss and for supporting overall health. While you are losing weight, toxins stored in the fat tissue are released into your bloodstream. Drinking plenty of pure water makes it easier for your liver and kidneys to eliminate toxins. Water also works with fiber to keep your bowels regular and prevent constipation. Feeling thirsty is a sign of dehydration, which is sometimes confused with hunger. Drinking water throughout the day will keep you hydrated and prevent dehydration.

Having a glass before and during meals can also help fill you up and reduce the quantity of food consumed. Add some lemon to your water with meals—the acidity of lemon will help lower the glycemic impact of your meal.

The National Research Council recommends that adults consume 4 cups of water for every 1,000 calories utilized by physical activity. If the average woman burns 2,200 calories per day, then she would need to drink 9 cups of water per day. You should consume more water if you are pregnant, breast-feeding, or engaging in vigorous physical exercise. Children should also try to drink at least 8 cups of water each day.

10. Choose Healthy, Low-GI Snacks and Desserts

There will always be times when you feel like something sweet or salty. You can enjoy a treat, just not every day. Get in the habit of reaching for fresh or dried fruit to satisfy sweet cravings. Carry low-GI snack bars with you, such as SoLo Gi bars, so that you won't be tempted by a candy bar. For dessert, your best options are a small piece of dark chocolate, frozen yogurt with baked apples and cinnamon, or a slice of flan cake. If you'd really like to have the double-fudge chocolate piece-of-heaven cheesecake, take a small portion and enjoy. For salt cravings, try a handful of nuts or seeds, or blue corn chips with hummus or feta dip. You can also experiment with different recipes to find a low-GI variation of your favorite dessert. You will likely find that as your body becomes accustomed to low-GI meals, you will have fewer cravings for high-GI foods and when you do eat them, you won't feel well. As a result, your desire for indulgence foods will decrease with time.

Glycemic Index Food Values Chart

On page 89 you will see a chart that shows you which foods are low, moderate, or high GI, based on GI testing done at the University of Sydney. Familiarize yourself with this chart and use it as a guide for shopping and meal preparation. Make a copy of this and put it on your fridge or carry it with you.

Here are some tips to help you lower the glycemic impact of your daily meals:

- Have at least one low-GI food at each meal.

- Pair the good with the bad: Combine a high-GI food with a low-GI food to reduce the overall glycemic impact of your meal.

- When eating high-GI foods, choose smaller portions.

- Don't indulge in excessive amounts of low-GI foods simply because they are low GI. Calories still count. While certain foods (ice cream, some chocolate bars, and french fries) might register as low GI, they should only be eaten in moderation or as an occasional treat because these foods are high in saturated fat and calories.

- Have quality protein and healthy fats with your carbs to reduce the glycemic impact.

- Eat sweets (desserts) after a meal rather than as a separate snack because after a meal, you will be full and satisfied with a smaller portion of a sweet. Also, having your sweets after a meal will have less of an impact on your blood sugar than having them on their own.

- Add lemon or vinegar to your meals as these acidic ingredients can significantly lower the glycemic impact of your meal.

- Use natural, alternative sweeteners such as stevia to sweeten foods such as cereal, yogurt, coffee, and whole-grain toast.

- Sprinkling cinnamon on your foods helps improve insulin sensitivity and blood sugar control.

- If you are diabetic, monitor your blood glucose level before eating and one to two hours afterward to see how different meal combinations impact your body. Keep a journal of what works for you and what doesn't.

Low Glycemic (55 or Less)	Moderate Glycemic (56–69)	High Glycemic (70 and over)
Apples (fresh and dried)	Arrowroot biscuit	Bagel (white)
Apple juice	Beer	Bread stuffing
Apricots (dried)	Beets (canned)	Broad beans
Banana (ripe)	Breton® crackers	Cereal (Cheerios™,
Barley	Buckwheat	Crispix™, Corn Flakes®,
Beans (haricot, lima,	Cantaloupe	Corn Pops®, Grapenuts™,
kidney, mung, navy,	Cereal (Shredded Wheat,	Rice, Krispies®, Total™)
and pinto)	Just Right, Nutrigrain, and	Corn cakes (puffed)
Bean sprouts	Raisin Bran	Corn chips, Dates
Broccoli	Corn (sweet)	Doughnut (cake type)
Carrots (raw)	Cornmeal	English muffin
Cereals (All-Bran™)	Couscous	French baguette
Chapati (bread)	Cranberry juice cocktail	French fries
Cherries	Croissant (white)	Fruit Roll-ups®
Chickpeas	Digestive biscuits	Glucose
Chocolate (dark)	Figs	Graham wafers
Grapefruit	Flan cake	Instant mashed potatoes
Grapes	Hamburger bun (white)	Jellybeans
Kiwi fruit	Honey	Kaiser roll
Lentils	Jam (strawberry)	Life Savers®
Milk	Mango (ripe)	Melba toast
Oat bran bread	Muesli	Pancake syrup
Oatmeal (slow-cook	Pancakes	Parsnips
oats)	Papaya	Pasta (corn, rice)
Oranges	Pasta (white, soft)	Popcorn
Pasta (al dente/firm)	Pineapple	Pop-Tarts™
Peaches (fresh and	Pita bread	Potato (baked)
dried)	Porridge (rolled oats)	Pretzels
Pears (fresh and dried)	Potatoes (mashed or	Rice (instant, jasmine,
Peppers	boiled)	sticky)
Plums	Raisins	Rice bread
Pumpernickel bread	Rice (basmati, brown)	Rice cakes (white)
Rice (long grain, con-	Rye bread	Rice crackers
verted, wild)	Split pea/green pea soup	Rutabagas
Sourdough bread	Sugar (sucrose)	Scone
Soybeans	Taco shells (corn)	Soda crackers
Soy beverages	Water crackers	Sports drinks
Split peas	Wheat Thins™	Tapioca (boiled)
Sushi	Whole wheat bread	Watermelon
Sweet potatoes		White bread
Syrup (pure maple)		
Taro		
Yam		
Yogurt (plain)		

Setting up Your Low-GI Home

It's easy to introduce a low-GI diet into your home without having to cook separate meals for different family members. This is a way of eating that is beneficial for everyone.

One of the biggest saboteurs of maintaining healthy eating habits is not having good food choices handy when you're rushed, stressed, and/or hungry, so I have listed some tips for shopping and stocking your pantry to get you started.

Shopping Low GI

- Instead of the traditional weekly bulk grocery trip, try to go shopping twice a week so that you can buy smaller amounts of fresh fruits and vegetables.

- Prepare your list ahead of time so that you know what you are buying and won't waste time wandering the aisles. Shop with certain meals in mind, which will help you steer clear of impulse purchases.

- Shop the perimeter of the grocery store, which is where the fresh foods are found. The center aisles stock the processed foods and snacks.

- Read labels and avoid products that contain sugar or refined flour in the first three ingredients. Also avoid products that contain trans fats (hydrogenated oils). Look for foods with a low GI rating—more products are being tested and rated all the time.

- Don't shop when you are hungry because you will tend to make impulse purchases and be tempted by the high-GI snacks and bakery items.

For the Refrigerator

The following items are great for eating nutritiously every day:

- Vegetables: Greens, yams, beans, broccoli, and carrots. Be sure to have lots of salad fixings on hand (lettuce, spinach, sprouts, peppers, and cucumbers)

- Fruits: Buy in season and eat when fresh

- 1 percent dairy products or fortified soy beverages
- Plain (unsweetened) yogurt
- Eggs (organic, omega-3 are best)
- Whole-grain breads such as rye, sourdough, pita, and flat bread
- Nut butters (almond and cashew)

Stocking Your Pantry

These staples are excellent to have on hand:

- Whole-grain flour (whole-wheat, rice, bran, and soy flour)
- Honey and pure maple syrup
- Whole-grain brown rice or wild rice
- Whole-wheat pasta
- Other grains such as quinoa, buckwheat, and couscous
- Beans (try to have three or four different types on hand as they are great in soups and stir-frys)
- Canned tomatoes, sugar-free tomato paste
- Canned salmon and tuna
- Low-GI cereals (try different brands to see what you like; don't be afraid to combine low- and moderate-GI cereals)
- Low-GI energy bars (such as SoLo Gi)
- Nuts and seeds (almonds, cashews, sunflower seeds, and flaxseeds)
- Slow-cook oatmeal
- Extra-virgin olive oil
- Dried spices
- Powdered cinnamon

Limit your intake of prepackaged foods, but stock frozen foods such as berries, vegetables, and lean meats—chicken, turkey, and fish, for example.

Holiday and Restaurant Survival Strategies

Following the glycemic index does not mean you've had your last restaurant or holiday feast meal. It's quite the opposite. Many diets are restrictive, which makes them difficult to follow. With the GI, you can continue to enjoy a variety of foods at home, parties, or in restaurants.

Here are some points to consider regarding restaurants and holidays:

1. Have a light, low-GI snack before you head out to a dinner party or restaurant so that you aren't tempted by high-GI appetizers.

2. Choose restaurants that offer a variety of freshly prepared foods. Avoid fast foods.

3. Experiment with international cuisine. Many foods found in Indian, Thai, Greek, and Japanese restaurants are naturally lower GI.

4. Don't be shy to ask questions. If you feel embarrassed, tell the waiter you are diabetic to ease the tension.

5. If you can't find a low-GI meal to your liking, order a half portion of the meal you would like, or see if the chef will make you a special dish.

6. Safe appetizers include: green salad with balsamic vinegar and olive oil, grilled vegetables, broiled scallops or shrimps, and pita bread with hummus or artichoke dip.

7. Limit alcohol consumption to no more than two glasses and also drink plenty of water with lemon.

8. Choose to have a glass of wine, or a whole-grain bread or bun, or dessert, but not all three. If you choose to have a bread or bun, be sure your main meal is primarily protein and vegetables. If you choose to have dessert, ask the chef which dessert is most appropriate for a low-GI diet. Some good options include berries or baked apples with frozen yogurt, dark chocolate or strawberry mousse, or flan.

9. To lower the GI of foods such as pasta, baked potatoes, or rice, you can open a capsule of Phase 2 and sprinkle it on the food before you eat it. Phase 2 reduces the breakdown of starch into sugar, thus lowering the glycemic impact of your meal.

10. If you are at a restaurant that serves large portions, ask for a take-out container when you order so that you don't overeat.

When planning holiday meals, don't be a slave to tradition, especially if traditional foods make you feel unwell. While there might be some temporary tastebud satisfaction, what counts is how you feel afterward. If what you eat haunts you afterward, whether through blood sugar swings, indigestion, or guilt, you should not be eating those foods. Instead, have fun creating your own holiday menu that includes fresh takes on classic dishes. For example, eat cauliflower or sweet potato mash instead of mashed potato, and instead of gravy thickened with corn starch, reach for different flavors of mustard and fresh or dried herbs. If you are dining at a friend's house and are concerned there won't be food choices for you, simply bring what you need.

Another concern with restaurant and holiday meals is that they often break the cycle of healthy eating habits. For people who struggle to establish consistent healthy eating habits, a break in the routine can be damaging on a larger scale, making it harder to get back on track. If you know this to be true about yourself, work hard to incorporate healthy GI choices at every meal. You will feel so proud of yourself and it will make it that much easier to continue on your path to success.

14-Day Meal Suggestions

The chart on the following pages provides a sample 14-day low-GI meal plan. It is not necessary to follow this exactly. It is simply a guideline. Feel free to make healthy substitutions. For example, if you are vegetarian, you will want to substitute the meat dishes with tofu, lentils, beans, and vegetables. Create meals that combine low- to moderate-GI carbs with protein and healthy fats. For a list of low-GI cookbooks, refer to the Resource section of this book. Remember to drink eight glasses or more of pure water each day. Herbal teas, especially green tea, are also encouraged.

	Breakfast	Snack	Lunch	Snack	Dinner
Saturday	2 whole-wheat pancakes with 1 tsp of real maple syrup and ½ cup of raspberries	1% cottage cheese with cucumber	Whole-wheat pasta sautéed with beans, tomato, and eggplant	1 pear	Green salad; small steak; sautéed onions and peppers; ½ cup of steamed beets; baked sweet potato
Friday	1 cup of plain yogurt with strawberries and 2 tbsp of ground flax or hemp; sprinkle with cinnamon	1 orange or ½ cup of cherries	Hummus with flatbread; salad with alfalfa sprouts, roasted peppers, and feta cheese	½ cup of trail mix	Green salad; grilled chicken with feta cheese, tomato, and avocado on sautéed spinach and carrots
Thursday	Power shake: Blend 1 scoop of protein powder with water, milk, or juice, plain yogurt, ice cubes, and berries	Low-GI energy bar	Egg salad on rye with lettuce, tomato, and cucumber; and an apple	cup of dried apricots	Green salad; grilled salmon with lemon; basmati rice; yellow squash and green beans
Wednesday	Egg white omelette (2 eggs) with feta cheese, spinach, and tomato; 1 slice of whole-grain toast with strawberry jam	¼ cup of almonds and an apple	Salmon sandwich on whole-wheat pita with lettuce and tomatoes; and red grapes	Low-GI energy bar	Green salad; chili (vegetarian or with meat); 1 small rye bun; ½ a cantaloupe
Tuesday	½ cantaloupe with sliced pears and plums, 1 low-GI energy bar (SoLo Gi)	½ cup of chickpeas, orange and red pepper	Lentil soup with corn tortilla, mixed green salad	¼ cup of almonds	Green salad; shrimp and scallops with whole-grain pasta and asparagus
Monday	Low-GI cereal such as All-Bran, skim or soy milk, and half a banana	Celery with cottage cheese	Crustless quiche (whole-grain flour, turkey, and broccoli)	1 apple with its skin	Green salad; sweet potato; turkey breast; green and yellow beans
Sunday	2 poached or scrambled eggs, turkey bacon, and 1 slice of pumpernickel or rye toast	1 cup of plain yogurt with blueberries	1 slice of pizza (whole-wheat crust, tomato sauce, 1% cheese, and chicken)	Carrot and celery sticks with yogurt	Green salad; grilled white fish; long-grain brown and wild rice with zucchini, onion, and, bok choy or Swiss chard

	Breakfast	Snack	Lunch	Snack	Dinner
Saturday	2 whole-wheat pancakes with 1 tsp of real maple syrup and ½ cup of blueberries	2 kiwi fruits	2 whole-wheat fajitas with grilled chicken, peppers, lettuce, tomato, low-fat cheese, and guacamole	Hummus with flatbread	Green salad; whole-wheat pasta stir-fry with soy sauce, tofu, almonds, and vegetables
Friday	Slow-cook oatmeal with dried apples, ground walnuts, and cinnamon	½ cup of cherries or berries with ½ cup of plain yogurt	Grilled chicken sandwich on rye with avocado, tomato, and lettuce; one pear	½ cup of trail mix	Green salad; grilled lamb cutlet with garlic; steamed carrots and green beans
Thursday	2 poached or scrambled eggs; 1 slice of whole-grain toast with almond butter	Low-GI energy bar	Pita bread stuffed with hummus, grilled eggplant, peppers, and tomato; an apple	2 oatmeal raisin cookies	Green salad; grilled tuna with soy sauce and ginger root; steamed brown rice; sautéed peppers, bean sprouts, and eggplant
Wednesday	Power shake: 1 scoop of protein powder with water/milk/juice, plain yogurt, ice cubes, and berries	4 whole-grain crackers with almond butter	2 corn or wheat tacos with lean ground turkey or beef, lettuce, tomato, salsa, and plain yogurt	Low-GI energy bar	Baked chicken with pineapple and ham; baked sweet potato; ½ a cantaloupe
Tuesday	2 whole-grain waffles with plain yogurt, berries, ground almonds, and cinnamon	¼ cup of cashews and an apple	Minestrone soup; 2 whole-grain crackers; ½ a cantaloupe	¼ cup of almonds	Green salad; whole-wheat pasta with tomato sauce, mushroom, peppers, onions, and lean beef
Monday	Slow-cook oatmeal with half a sliced mango, flaxseed, and cinnamon; ½ cup of plain yogurt	Low-GI energy bar	Greek salad (lettuce, tomato, olives, and feta cheese); grilled chicken breast	Pear with skin	Green salad; grilled salmon with lemon and dill; brown rice and steamed broccoli
Sunday	Egg-white omelette (2 eggs) with asparagus, onion, and cottage cheese; ½ slice of whole-grain toast	1 cup of plain yogurt with muesli	Pasta salad with grilled eggplant, peppers, and mushrooms; ½ a mango	Carrot and celery sticks with yogurt	Green salad; grilled pork chops; baked sweet potato; sautéed spinach; dark chocolate mousse

Five Keys to Success

1. Don't look at this as a diet. It is a healthy way of eating that will make you feel and look better. There are lots of great low- and moderate-GI foods that you can enjoy, and it is okay to have high-GI foods too—just mix them with low-GI foods. Experiment and have fun trying new low-GI recipes (recommended cookbooks are in the back of this book).

2. Be physically active at least five days a week, every week. Don't make excuses not to exercise. Instead, give yourself reasons why you like to exercise, such as you like having more energy, better sleep, and a better mood. If weather conditions are keeping you indoors, turn on the radio or put in a CD and work out inside.

3. Get adequate sleep at night and find ways to minimize your stress level. Remember these two factors can impact appetite, cravings, and many other bodily processes.

4. Be smart about your supplements. Choose clinically tested supplements to support your blood sugar management and weight-loss efforts, such as fiber, Phase 2, and CLA.

5. Make an effort to have a positive attitude and to be kind to yourself. This is the hardest of all because you may have tried other diets in the past and failed. Stay positive and optimistic. Work on overcoming negative thinking and celebrate every success, especially during the transition. For each week you maintain your diet and exercise routine, treat yourself to something very special, like a new CD or outfit. You will have earned it.

Setting Manageable Goals

Health authorities agree that in order to maintain long-term weight loss, you need to make long-term changes to your lifestyle. Rather than looking for a quick fix, work on developing a comprehensive strategy that includes a balanced, low-glycemic diet, consistent exercise, and safe supplements.

When you're ready to do it, you need to make a commitment to lifelong changes. Changing your diet and lifestyle for a few weeks is a great start, but it is not enough to reduce your risk of disease and increase your lifelong vitality. For long-term success, you need to make long-term changes. Start by setting some reasonable goals for yourself. Trying to change too many things at once can set you up for frustration and failure. Instead, try to make one or two changes each week. For example, one change could be to substitute white bread/pasta/rice for brown. Another could be to cut down or cut out soft drinks and switch to herbal teas. Next, try eating more frequent and smaller meals rather than three larger meals. The same holds for exercise. Gradually increase the time, intensity, and frequency of your workouts so that your body can adjust. While you may be excited and eager to make a lot of changes to your lifestyle, I suggest setting reasonable goals that you can attain and incorporating your changes gradually.

Remember, it took a lifetime to develop your current habits, so they won't disappear overnight. This will be a work in progress that may take as long as a year to fall into a comfortable rhythm. Consider the first three months as the transition time:

- Month One is your adjustment period. Be kind to yourself and experiment as much as possible as you adjust from your old way of eating to your new way.

- Month Two should see this new way of eating become a habit. During this month, be disciplined about sticking to your new eating habits. Discover where you have challenges, such as being too busy on weeknights to cook, and develop strategies to deal with these challenges.

ॐ During Month Three you should start to see noticeable improvements to your health, blood sugar, and weight. Otherwise seek expert advice.

If you're not making headway by the end of Month Three, consider hiring a professional to get some guidance on moving in the right direction.

ॐ *Registered dietitian:* Book an appointment with a registered dietitian to help identify your problem areas and learn strategies to overcome them. It may take no more than one appointment to get things straightened out. Keep a food journal before your first appointment.

ॐ *Naturopath (or complementary health care provider):* A holistic health care provider can work with you to identify problems such as nutritional deficiencies or food allergies that may be impacting your ability to lose weight and stick to a new eating style.

ॐ *Counselor:* If your relationship with food seems like it's not in your control, you may be suffering from compulsive or emotional eating. Expert advice could help you overcome this obstacle.

Brace for Impact

Be prepared for some rocky roads during the transition to low-GI foods. While in only a short period of time you should start to feel better, most notably with more balanced mood, increased energy, and better digestion, you could also have some temporary side effects from the change of diet such as headaches, fatigue, irritability, and cravings. This is your body telling you that it wants a blood sugar boost *now*. If you are going to overcome food cravings and take control of your blood sugar, you will have to suffer through these difficult times. (However, please consult your physician if these side effects last longer than a week.) If you can make it through the transition period and get your diet on the right track, with balanced blood sugar instead of blood sugar highs and lows, you will begin to feel well, energized, and more in control of what you eat. In the meantime, reach for an apple, an orange pepper, a small amount of dried fruit and nuts, or yogurt and berries.

You may also feel self-conscious about being a "high-maintenance" or "fussy" eater. In some cases, coworkers, friends, or family may make unkind comments about your new habits. You may experience some peer pressure to not "rock the boat" and to eat what everyone else is eating. Take heart. This just comes with the territory of eating outside the typical (and unhealthy) diet, so you better learn to ignore it. Remember that nobody else is living your life. You have only one chance and you need to make the most of it, and that includes feeling your best every day. Obesity and diabetes can make you feel lousy and take years off your life. Remind yourself of the end goal when you're faced with insensitive comments. Just smile to yourself and shrug them off, knowing that you are doing what's best for your health.

————•◦•◦•————

An English proverb says, "Don't dig your own grave with a knife and fork." As you have read in this book, there are many health concerns associated with a high-GI diet—concerns that can diminish quality of life and shorten your life span.

Improving our eating habits is the long-term answer to many health concerns we face. Making the change to a low-GI diet offers a number of benefits. This sensible and health-conscious eating style has proven benefits for weight loss, appetite control, and blood sugar management. Numerous studies have also shown that a low-GI diet can help protect against two of the major health threats that we face, namely, diabetes and heart disease. This is a safe way of eating for children, teenagers, pregnant women, nursing moms, seniors, and anyone interested in better health.

It is my sincere hope that you will take what you've learned from this book and put it into action in your life. I am confident that if you put the time and effort into following a low-GI diet, combined with regular exercise and proper sleep and stress-management strategies, you will see tremendous results for your overall health. I wish you the best of luck as you set forth on your path to weight-loss success.

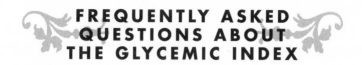

FREQUENTLY ASKED QUESTIONS ABOUT THE GLYCEMIC INDEX

What is the difference between the glycemic index (GI) and the glycemic load (GL)?

The glycemic index is a ranking of how fast and how much a carbohydrate containing food affects blood glucose levels. It is measured using a standardized serving of a food that provides 50 grams of carbohydrate. For example, three apples provide 50 grams of carbohydrate so this is the amount used to determine the GI of apples. All foods are compared to glucose, which has a value of 100. Foods that have a value of 55 or less are considered low GI, those that rank between 56 and 69 are moderate, and those with values above 70 are considered high GI. The GL tells us how a particular serving of that food will affect our blood glucose levels. It is calculated by multiplying the GI of the food by the amount of carbohydrates (in grams) in your serving and dividing by 100. For example, most people eat one apple rather than three as a serving. The GI of apples is 34 and there are about 15 grams of carbohydrate in one average apple. The GL is therefore 34 times 15 divided by 100, which equals 5. Foods with a GL of 10 or less are considered low, those with a GL between 11 and 19 are considered moderate, and those with a GL of greater than 20 are considered high.

Why do some foods not appear in the GI list?

The GI is relevant only for carbohydrate foods. Foods that contain little or no carbohydrate, such as meat, fish, eggs, nuts, and seeds, cannot be tested for the GI.

What is the GI of alcoholic beverages?

Alcoholic beverages (wine and spirits) contain very little carbohydrate unless they are mixed with juices or soda pop. Beer contains some carbohydrate—a 10-ounce glass has about 10 grams of carbohydrate compared with 36 grams in the same volume of soft drink. For this reason, a beer will raise glucose levels slightly. If you drink a large amount of beer, then it will have a more significant effect on blood glucose. It is okay to have a drink or two per day, but keep in mind that alcohol floods the body with empty calories.

Can you eat too many low-GI foods?

Yes. Even if a food has a low GI ranking, you need to exercise portion control as calories still count. Excess calories, whether they come from carbohydrate, protein, or fat, can be stored in the body as fat. Overeating on a regular basis can not only lead to weight problems, but it can also increase the risk of chronic diseases and shorten your life span. Small portions, on the other hand, have been linked to a healthier lifestyle and greater longevity.

Why does rice have so many different GI values?

There are many factors that affect the GI of a food, such as the type of starch, the fiber content, and how it is processed and cooked. There are several types of rice (white, brown, red, black, long-grain, short-grain, instant, converted, and sticky rice, for example) and they vary in their ratio of the starches amylose and amylopectin and their fiber content. The more amylose and fiber in a rice, the lower the GI. For example, long-grain brown rice has more fiber and more amylose compared to short-grain white rice, and thus has a much lower GI.

Should diabetics avoid high-GI vegetables?

Absolutely not. Vegetables contain a very low amount of carbohydrate, so even though some are high GI, their glycemic load is low. Vegetables provide us with essential vitamins, minerals, and fiber. Eat a variety of vegetables to ensure that you get the wide range of nutrients that they provide.

Why is the GI of potato chips and french fries lower than that of baked potatoes?

Large amounts of fat in a food will slow the rate of stomach emptying and therefore the rate of digestion, leading to a lower impact on blood glucose levels. High-fat foods, such as potato chips and other fried foods, are not better for you because they have a lower GI. These foods are high in calories, and eating a diet high in saturated and trans fats is associated with increased risk of heart disease and certain cancers. Keep in mind the GI is meant to be used in conjunction with other healthy eating principles.

Most breads and bagels are high GI. Should I avoid them?

White bread and baked goods made with white flour are high GI and should be avoided because they lack nutritional value and have a strong impact on blood glucose levels. However, you can enjoy high-fiber breads, rye bread, and pumpernickel breads, which are low to moderate GI, in your daily diet.

Is brown sugar lower in the GI than white sugar?

No, brown sugar is moderate GI, which is the same as white sugar. Brown sugar is brown in color because it is coated with molasses syrup. It is not any better for you, or lower in the GI, compared to white sugar.

Where do sugar substitutes fall in the glycemic index?

Artificial sweeteners such as aspartame and saccharin do not have a high glycemic index because they are not carbohydrates. Splenda (sucralose) is another artificial sweetener that does contain some calories and has a GI rating because it contains maltodextrin, which is high GI. Until more is known about the long-term affects of consuming foods and beverages containing these artificial ingredients, I would recommend avoiding or minimizing their use. Instead, consider using stevia, which is a natural plant sweetener that is about 300 times sweeter than sugar, without the calories or impact on blood glucose levels.

Is a low-GI diet safe for children or the elderly?

Yes, a low-GI diet is a healthy way of eating that does not exclude carbohydrates or any other food group. It just involves making healthier carbohydrate choices. A low-GI diet can help improve a number of health parameters, such as blood glucose levels, cholesterol, and body weight. People also find that they have more energy, fewer mood swings, and better concentration throughout the day.

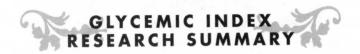

GLYCEMIC INDEX RESEARCH SUMMARY

*S*ince the 1981 publication of the University of Toronto research paper that gave us the term liglycemic index, there has been a great deal of scientific study about the benefits of low-GI foods. The studies have a common goal: They want to further understand the glycemic response and to document what benefits the varying responses might produce to prevent chronic diseases such as obesity, type 2 diabetes, heart disease, and cancer. Canada's University of Toronto and Australia's University of Sydney are leading research hubs on the glycemic index, but there are also ongoing studies around the world. Here is a sampling of compelling published research to date:

In a 2006 study published in the Archives of Internal Medicine, researchers from the University of Sydney proved that low glycemic load diets reduce blood glucose and insulin levels. In this 12-week controlled study, 129 overweight or obese people were randomly assigned one of four diets:

- ❧ High carbohydrate/low glycemic load
- ❧ High carbohydrate/high glycemic load
- ❧ High protein, carb reduced/ low glycemic load
- ❧ High protein, carb reduced/ high glycemic load

The participants were given calorie-restricted meal plans and access to a dietician. Due to calorie restrictions, all four diets resulted in weight loss of between 4 and 6 percent. However, the high carbohydrate/low glycemic index diet produced the best outcome, reducing both body fat and LDL (bad cholesterol). The diet that was high carbohydrate and high glycemic was associated with the slowest rate of weight loss. In the high carbohydrate diets, but not the high protein diet, lowering the glycemic load doubled the amount of body fat lost. The researchers concluded that even moderate reductions in glycemic load increase the rate of body fat loss, particularly for women. (Archives of Internal Medicine 2006; 166: 1466–1475).

In a 1999 issue of *Pediatrics*, a group of researchers from Tufts University in Boston reported a relationship between a high-glycemic diet, overeating, and obesity. They evaluated the food intake of 12 obese teenage boys after three separate meals (low GI, moderate GI, and high GI), and found that the boys consumed significantly more food after a moderate-GI and high-GI meal than after a low-GI meal. The researchers concluded, *"The rapid absorption of glucose after consumption of high GI meals induces a sequence of hormonal and metabolic changes that promote excessive food intake in obese subjects."* (Pediatrics, 1999 Mar;103(3): E26)

Research published in *Diabetes Care* in 2000 found that high blood glucose levels or repeated glycemic "spikes" following a meal may promote type 2 diabetes and coronary heart disease by increasing oxidative damage to the cardiovascular system and also by directly increasing insulin levels. *(Diabetes Care 2000 Dec; 23(12):1830–4)*

In 2002, the University of Toronto partnered with researchers in France and Sweden and published an overview on the glycemic index. They said, "The glycemic index has particular relevance to those chronic Western diseases associated with central obesity and insulin resistance.... sufficient, positive findings have emerged to suggest that the dietary glycemic index is of potential importance in the treatment and prevention of chronic diseases. *(American Journal of Clinical Nutrition 2002; 76: 266S–73S)*

Also in 2002, published in the *European Journal of Clinical Nutrition,* a group of researchers from Toronto, France, and Italy looked at the scientific evidence and role of the glycemic index on chronic Western disease. They found several health benefits exist for reducing the rate of carbohydrate absorption by means of a low-GI diet, including reduced insulin demand, improved blood glucose control, and reduced blood lipid levels. *(European Journal of Clinical Nutrition 54:353–355*

In 2004, a study revealed that high insulin levels, or a high sugar diet (which causes high insulin levels), are connected with a higher incidence of prostate cancer. (*Journal of Cancer* 2004;112: 446). It was shown in a previous study that increased insulin levels are associated with more advanced prostate cancer (*British Journal of Cancer* 2002; 87: 726).

In 2004, a prospective study by Canadian researchers in the *International Journal of Cancer* (2005; 114(4): 653–658) found that post-menopausal women with high overall dietary glycemic index values were at increased risk of breast cancer. A prospective study in the United States found that premenopausal women with high overall dietary glycemic index values and low levels of physical activity were also at increased risk of breast cancer (*Cancer Epidemiology Biomarkers & Prevention* 2004;13(1):65–70).

According to articles in the *Journal of the National Cancer Institute* (2002; 94:1293–1300 and 2004; 96(3): 229-233) some studies suggest increased risk of colorectal cancer with a high-glycemic diet.

In 2005, the *American Journal of Clinical Nutrition* published a report that found that study participants lost more weight on a "slow carb" or low-glycemic-load diet than on a low-fat or low-carb diet. After 12 months on the various diets, the slow-carb group lost 7.8 percent of their body weight compared with 6.1 percent in the low-fat-diet group. The levels of triglycerides (blood fats linked to heart disease) were also decreased by 37 percent in the slow-carb group versus 19 percent in the low-fat group. *(American Journal of Clinical Nutrition 2005; 81: 976–982)*

————•◦•◦•————

There is no shortage of research on the GI. If you would like to read about more studies, visit: www.glycemicindex.com. This is the "Home of the Glycemic Index," run by the Human Nutrition Unit, School of Molecular and Microbial Biosciences at the University of Sydney and top glycemic index expert Professor Jennie Brand-Miller. Each month, the site offers a free e-newsletter with research updates as well as lifestyle and diet tips. This is a terrific resource to stay informed on glycemic index research. The Glycemic Research Institute in Washington, DC, on the web at www. glycemic.com, is also another valuable resource for up-to-date research on the glycmic index.

RECOMMENDED READING AND RESOURCES

Recommended Reading

Brand-Miller, Dr. Jennie, and Kaye Foster-Powell with Joanna McMillan-Price. *The Low GI Diet Revolution.* New York City: Marlowe & Company, 2005.

Burani, Johanna. *Good Carbs, Bad Carbs: Lose Weight and Enjoy Optimum Health and Vitality by Eating the Right Carbs.* New York City: Marlowe & Company, 2004.

Canadian Diabetes Association. *Beyond the Basics.* Toronto: Canadian Diabetes Association, 2006.

Graci, Sam. *The Path to Phenomenal Health.* Toronto: John Wiley & Sons, 2005.

Karst, Karlene. *The Metabolic Syndrome Program: How to Lose Weight, Beat Heart Disease, Stop Insulin Resistance, and More.* Toronto: John Wiley & Sons, 2006.

King, Brad. *Awaken Your Metabolism: Your Ultimate Guide to Abundant Energy.* Hillsburg: Health Venture Publications, 2005.

Murray, Michael, ND. *How to Prevent and Treat Diabetes with Natural Medicine.* New York City: Riverhead Books, 2004.

Preuss, Harry. *The Natural Fat Loss Pharmacy.* New York City: Broadway, 2007.

Low-GI Cookbooks

Brand-Miller, Dr. Jennie, Kaye Foster-Powell, Kate Marsh, and Philippa Sandell. *The New Glucose Revolution Low GI Vegetarian Cookbook: 80 Delicious Vegetarian and Vegan Recipes Made Easy with the Glycemic Index.* New York City: Marlowe & Company, 2006.

Brand-Miller, Dr. Jennie, Kate Foster-Powell, and Joanna McMillan-Price. *The Low GI Diet Cookbook: 100 Simple, Delicious Smart-Carb Recipes-The Proven Way to Lose Weight and Eat for Lifelong Health.* New York City: Marlowe & Company, 2005.

Brand-Miller, Dr. Jennie, Hill, Rachael Anne, and Nicki Dowey. *GI High-Energy Cookbook: Low-GI Recipes for Weight Loss, Health and Vitality.* New York City: Ryland Peters and Small, 2006.

Maar, Nancy T. *The Everything Glycemic Index Cookbook: 300 Appetizing Recipes to Keep Your Weight Down and Your Energy Up!* Avon: Adams Media, 2006.

Helpful Resources

For information on the glycemic index and healthy eating:
Glycemic Research Institute: www.glycemic.com
Harvard School of Public Health, The Nutrition Source:
www.hsph.harvard. edu/nutritionsource
University of Sydney, official site of the Glycemic Index:
www.glycemicindex.com

For information on diabetes:
American Diabetes Association: www.diabetes.org
Canadian Diabetes Association: www.diabetes.ca
Diabetes UK: www.diabetes.org/uk
International Diabetes Institute (Australia): www.diabetes.com.au

For general information on herbs, vitamins, and nutritional supplements:

www.healthwell.com

www.iherb.com

Linus Pauling Institute: lpi.oregonstate.edu

www.pdrhealth.com

www.wholehealthmd.com

For information on the products discussed in this book:

Advantra Z®: www.nutratechinc.com

PGX™: www.slimstyles.com

Phase 2® Starch Neutralizer: www.phase2info.com

Tonalin® CLA: www.tonalin.com

Other health links:

American College of Sports Medicine: http://acsm.org/index.asp

American Heart Association Fitness Resource: www.justmove.org

Author's Web site: www.sherrytorkos.com

Centers for Disease Control and Prevention: www.cdc.gov

Institute of Medicine: www.iom.edu

Mayo Clinic: www.mayoclinic.com

National Institutes of Health: www.nih.gov

National Institutes of Health, Calculate your BMI:
www.nhlbisupport.com/bmi/

Reuters Health (for the latest medical and health care news):
www.reutershealth.com

Web MD: www.webmd.com

Product Directory

The supplements for weight loss and blood sugar control listed in this book are available under the following brands:

Advantra Z®

Bitter Orange by Nature's Way®

Cortislim® Original™ and Cortislim® Burn™ by Window Rock
   Enterprises, Inc.
Diet Fuel® and Ripped Fuel® by Twin Lab®
Green Tea Fat Burner® by Applied Nutrition®
Lean System 7® by iSotori
Look Slim by Prolab®

PGX™

BodySense® Meal Replacement with PGX® by Preferred Nutrition
METAslim No Nonsense Diet™ by WN Pharmaceuticals® Ltd.
Slim Styles™ by Natural Factors®

Phase 2®

BodySense® Natural Diet Program by Preferred Nutrition
CARB CUTTER Phase 2® by Health & Nutrition Systems
   International, Inc.
METASlim Carb Neutralizer & Fat Blocker, METASlim Phase 2®,
   and METASlim Kit by WN Pharmaceuticals® Ltd.
Phase 2® by Nature's Harmony®, NOW® Foods, Vivitas™,
   Slenderite™, and Carb Intercept® by Natrol®
Total Lean Advance™ by General Nutrition Centers Inc.
TRIMSPA® CarbSpa by Nutramerica Corporation

Tonalin® CLA

Tonalin® CLA is available by Country Life®, General Nutrition
   Centers Inc., Jarrow Formulas®, Natrol®, Natural Factors®,
   Nature's Bounty®, Nature's Way®, Preferred Nutrition®, Swiss
   Herbal Remedies, and WN Pharmaceuticals® Ltd.

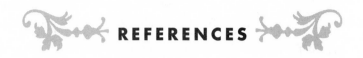# REFERENCES

Augustin, L.S., Galeone, C., Dal Maso, L., et al. "Glycemic index, glycemic load, and risk of prostate cancer." *Int J Cancer* 112 (2004): 446.

Ballerini, R. "Evaluation of efficacy and safety of a food supplement for weight control through the reduced-calories intake from carbohydrates vs. placebo." Data on file. Pharmachem Laboratories, Kearny, New Jersey, 2002.

Bell, S.J., Sears, B. "Low-glycemic-load diets: Impact on obesity and chronic diseases." *Crit Rev Food Sci Nutr.* 43, no. 4 (2003): 357–377.

Birmingham, C.L., Muller, J.L., Palepn, A., Spinelli, J.J., and Anise, A.H. "Cost of obesity in Canada." *CMAJ* 160 (1999): 483–488.

Blankson, H., Stakkestad, J.A., Fagertun, H., et al. "Conjugated linoleic acid reduces body fat mass in overweight and obese humans." *J Nutr* 130, no. 12 (2000): 2943–2948.

Boule, N.G., Haddad, E., Kenny, G.P., Wells, G.A., and Sigal, R.J. "Effects of exercise on glycemic control and body mass in type 2 diabetes mellitus: A meta-analysis of controlled clinical trials." *JAMA* 286, no. 10 (2001): 1218–1227.

Brehm, B.J., Seeley, R.J., Daniels, S.R., et al. "A randomized trial comparing a very low-carbohydrate diet and a calorie-restricted low-fat diet on body weight and cardiovascular risk factors in healthy women." *J Clin Endocrinol Metab* 88, no. 4 (2003): 1617–1623.

Carmona, Richard H. M.D., M.P.H., F.A.C.S., Surgeon General, U.S. Public Health Service, U.S. Department of Health and Human Services. Statements made before the Subcommittee on Competition, Infrastructure, and Foreign Commerce Committee on Commerce, Science, and Transportation United States Senate, released March 2, 2004.

Chantre, P., and Lairon, D. "Recent findings of green tea extract AR25 (Exolise) and its activity for the treatment of obesity." *Phytomedicine* 9 (2002): 3–8.

Chaoyang, L., Ford, E.S., Mokdad, A.H., et al. "Recent trends in waist circumference and waist-height ratio among US children and adolescents." *Pediatrics* 118 (2006): e1391–e1398.

Colker, C.M., et al. "Effects of citrus aurantium extract, caffeine, and St. John's wort on body fat loss, lipid levels, and mood states in overweight healthy adults." *Curr Ther Res* 60 (1999): 145–153.

Cunningham, Dr. Sam, et al. "Managing glycemic response." *Nutraceuticals World* (September 20, 2006)

Dansinger, M.L., Gleason, J.L., Griffith, J.L., et al. "One year effectiveness of the Atkins, Ornish, Weight Watchers, and Zone diets in decreasing body weight and heart disease risk." Presented at the American Heart Association Scientific Sessions, November 12, 2003, Orlando.

DeLany, J.P., Blohm, E., Truett, A.A., et al. "Conjugated linoleic acid rapidly reduces body fat content in mice without affecting energy intake." *Am J Physiol* 276 (1999): 1172–1179.

Diabetes and Nutrition Study Group (DNSG) of the European Association for the Study of Diabetes (EASD). "Recommendations for the nutritional management of patients with diabetes mellitus." *Eur J Clin Nutr* 54 (2000): 353–355.

Dulloo, A.G., et al. "The thermogenic properties of ephedrine/methylxantine mixtures 11: human studies." *Int J Obes* 10 (1986): 467–481.

Dulloo, A.G., Duret, C., Rohrer, D., et al. "Efficacy of a green tea extract rich in catechin polyphenols and caffeine in increasing 24-h energy expenditure and fat oxidation in humans." *Am J Clin Nutr* 70 (1999): 1040–1045.

Ebbeling, C.B., Leidig, M.M., Sinclair, K.B., et al. "Effects of an ad libitum low-glycemic load diet on cardiovascular disease risk factors in obese young adults." *Am Journal Clin Nutr* 81 (2005): 976–982.

Flier, J.S. "Obesity." In *Joslin's Diabetes Mellitus*, 13th ed., edited by R.C. Kahn and G.C. Weir, 351–361. Philadelphia: Lea & Febiger, 1994.

Foster, G.D., Wyatt, H.R., Hill, J.O., et al. "A randomized trial of a low-carbohydrate diet for obesity." *N Engl J Med* 348, no. 21 (2003): 2082–2090.

Foster-Powell, K., Holt, S.H., and Brand-Miller, J.C. "International table of glycemic index and glycemic load values." *Am J Clin Nutr.* 76 (2002): 5–56.

Franz, M.J., Bantle, and J.P., Beebe, C.A. "Evidence-based nutrition principles and recommendations for the treatment and prevention of diabetes and related complications." *Diabetes Care* 2002: 148–198.

Gasteyger, C., and Tremblay, A. "Metabolic impact of body fat distribution." *J Endocrinol Invest* 25 (2002): 876–883.

Gaullier, J.M., Halse, J., Hoye, K., et al. "Conjugated linoleic acid supplementation for 1 y reduces body fat mass in healthy overweight humans." *Am J Clin Nutr* 79 (2004): 1118–1125.

Haffner, S.M. "Epidemiological studies on the effects of hyperglycemia and improvement of glycemic control on macrovascular events in type 2 diabetes." *Diabetes Care* 22, no. 3, Supplement (1999): 54–56.

Health Canada. Canadian Community Health Survey, 2004. Accessed November 23, 2006. Available online at: http://www.hc-sc.gc.ca/fn-an/surveill/nutrition/commun/index_e.html.

Higginbotham, S., Zhang, Z.F., Lee, I.M., et al. "Dietary glycemic load and risk of colorectal cancer in the Women's Health Study." *J Natl Cancer Inst* 96, no. 3 (2004): 229–233.

Higginbotham, S., Zhang, Z.F., Lee, I.M., Cook, N.R., Buring, J.E., and Liu, S. "Dietary glycemic load and breast cancer risk in the Women's Health Study." *Cancer Epidemiol Biomarkers Prev* 13, no. 1 (2004): 65–70.

Institute of Medicine of the National Academies. "Dietary reference intakes for energy, carbohydrate, fiber, fat, fatty acids, cholesterol, protein, and amino acids." Accessed October 24, 2006. Available online at: www.iom.edu.

Jenkins, D.J., Kendall, C.W., Augustin, L.S., et al. "Glycemic index: Overview of implications in health and disease." *Am J Clin Nutr* 76 (2002): 266S–273S.

King, A.C., et al. "Moderate-intensity exercise and self-rated quality of sleep in older adults: A randomized controlled trial." *JAMA* 277 (1997): 32–37.

Kings Fund Policy Institute. "Counting the cost: The real impact of non-insulin dependent diabetes." A Kings Fund Report commissioned by the British Diabetic Association, London, 1996.

Kramer, F.M., et al. "Long-term follow-up of behavioural treatment of obesity: Patterns of regain among men and women." *Intl J Obesity* 13 (1989): 123–126.

Kushi, L.H., Fee, R.M., Folsom, A.R., et al. "Physical activity and mortality in postmenopausal women." *JAMA* 277, no. 16 (1997): 1287–1292.

Lean, M.E., et al. "Waist circumference as a measure for indicating need for weight management." *BMJ* 311 (1995): 158–161.

Lehrer, S., Diamond, E.J., Stagger, S., et al. "Serum insulin level, disease stage, prostate specific antigen (PSA) and Gleason score in prostate cancer." *Br J Cancer* 87, no. 7 (2002): 726–728.

Liese, A.D., Roach, A.K., Sparks, K.C., et al. "Whole-grain intake and insulin sensitivity: The Insulin Resistance Atherosclerosis Study." *Am J Clin Nutr* 78 (2003): 965–971.

Ludwig, D.S. "Dietary glycemic index and obesity." *J Nutr* 130 (2000): 280S–283S.

Ludwig, D.S., Majzoub, Joseph A., Al-Zahrani, Ahmed, et al. "High glycemic index foods, overeating, and obesity." *Pediatrics* 103, no. 3 (1999): e26.

Lynch, J., et al. "Moderately intense physical activities and high levels of cardiorespiratory fitness reduce the risk of non-insulin-dependent diabetes mellitus in middle-aged men." *Arch Intern Med* 156 (1996): 1307–1314.

MacDonald, H.B. "Conjugated linoleic acid and disease prevention: A review of current knowledge." *J Am Coll Nutr* 19, no. 2 (2000): 11S–118S.

Madrick, B. "Carbohydrate counting." Toronto: Canadian Diabetes Association, June 16, 2002.

Manson, J.E., et al. "Body weight and mortality." *N Engl J Med* 333 (1995): 677–685.

McMillan-Price, J., Petocz, P., Atkinson, F., et al. "Comparison of 4 diets of varying glycemic load on weight loss and cardiovascular risk reduction in overweight and obese young adults: A randomised controlled trial." *Arch Intern Med.* 166 (2006): 1466–1475.

Mendis, Shanthi, et al. "Integrated management of cardiovascular risk." Report of a World Health Organization meeting, Geneva, July 2002.

Michaud, D.S., Liu, S., Giovannucci, E., Willett, W.C., Colditz, G.A., and Fuchs, C.S. "Dietary sugar, glycemic load, and pancreatic cancer risk in a prospective study." *J Natl Cancer Inst* 94, no. 17 (2002): 1293–1300.

Mokdad, A.H., Bowman, B.A., Ford, E.S., Vinicor, F., Marks, J.S., and Koplan, J.P. "The continuing epidemics of obesity and diabetes in the United States." *JAMA* 286, no. 10 (2001): 1195–2000.

National Institute of Diabetes and Digestive and Kidney Diseases. *Understanding Adult Obesity.* NIH Publication, no. 94-3680. Rockville: National Institutes of Health, 1993.

National Institutes of Health. "Consensus conference on methods for voluntary weight loss and control." *Ann Int Med* 116 (1992): 942–949.

North American Society for the Study of Obesity's Annual Scientific Meeting, Las Vegas, November 14–18, 2004. WebMD Medical News: "Sleep more and you may control eating more." WebMD Medical News: "Why dieting makes you hungrier." News release, North American Society for the Study of Obesity.

Organization for Economic Co-operation and Development (OECD) Health Data 2006: A comparative analysis of 30 countries. Accessed November 23, 2006. Available online at: http://www.oecd.org/health/healthdata/

Organization for Economic Co-operation and Development (OECD). "Obesity and Health Forum 2004." Presented by John P. Martin, May 12, 2004.

Office of the Surgeon General. "Overweight and obesity: The Surgeon General's call to action to prevent and decrease overweight and obesity," December, 2001. Accessed November 23, 2006. Available online at: http://www.surgeongeneral.gov/topics/obesity.

Park, Y., Albright, K.J., Liu, W., et al. "Effect of conjugated linoleic acid on body composition in mice." *Lipids* 32, no. 8 (1997): 853–858.

Park, Y., Albright, K.J., Storkson, J.M., et al. "Changes in body composition in mice during feeding and withdrawal of conjugated linoleic acid." *Lipids* 34, no. 3 (1998): 243–248.

Pelkman, C.L. "Effects of the glycemic index of foods on serum concentrations of high-density lipoprotein cholesterol and triglycerides." *Curr Atheroscler Rep* 3, no. 6 (2001): 456–461.

Pereira, M.A., and Liu, S. "Types of carbohydrates and risk of cardiovascular disease." *J Women's Health* 12 (2003): 115–122.

Pi-Sunyer, F.X., et al. "Medical hazards of obesity." *Ann Intern Med* 119 (1993): 655–660.

Reaven, G. "The insulin resistance syndrome: Past, present, and future." Presented at the First Annual World Congress on the Insulin Resistance Syndrome, November 20–22, 2003, Los Angeles.

Riserus, U., Berglund, L., and Vessby, B. "Conjugated linoleic acid (CLA) reduced abdominal adipose tissue in obese middle-aged men with signs of the metabolic syndrome: A randomised controlled trial." *Int J Obes Relat Metah Disord* 25, no. 8 (August 2001): 1129–1135.

Schulze, M.B., Liu, S., Rimm, E.B., et al. "Glycemic index, glycemic load, and dietary fiber intake and incidence of type 2 diabetes in younger and middle-aged women." *Am J Clin Nutr* 80 (2004): 348–356.

Shrier, I. "Stretching before exercise: An evidence-based approach." *Br J Sports Med* 34, no. 5 (2000): 324–325.

Silvera, S.A., Jain, M., Howe, G.R., Miller, A.B., and Rohan, T.E. "Dietary carbohydrates and breast cancer risk: A prospective study of the roles of overall glycemic index and glycemic load." *Int J Cancer* 114, no. 4 (2005): 653–658.

Smedman, A., and Vessby, B. "Conjugated linoleic acid supplementation in humans—metabolic effects." *Lipids* 36, no. 8 (2001): 773–781.

Steinberger, J., and Daniels, S.R. "Obesity, insulin resistance, diabetes, and cardiovascular risk in children." *Circulation* 107 (2003): 1448.Temel-kova-Kurktschiev, T.S., Koehler, C., Henkel, E., et al. "Postchallenge plasma glucose and glycemic spikes are more strongly associated with atherosclerosis than fasting glucose or HbA1c level." *Diabetes Care* 23, no. 12 (2000): 1830–1834.

Thom, E. "A pilot study with the aim of studying the efficacy and tolerability of Tonalin CLA on the body composition in humans." Medstat Research Ltd., Lillestrom, Norway, 1997.

Van Gaal, L.F., Mertens, I.L., and Ballaux, D. "What is the relationship between risk factor reduction and degree of weight loss?" *Eur Heart J* 7, no. 50, Supplement (2005): L21–L26.

Wolever, T.M., Yang, M., Zeng, X.Y., et al. "Food glycemic index, as given in glycemic index tables, a significant determinant of glycemic responses elicited by composite breakfast meals." *Am J Clin Nutr* 83 (2006): 1306–1312.

DEC 0 6 2007